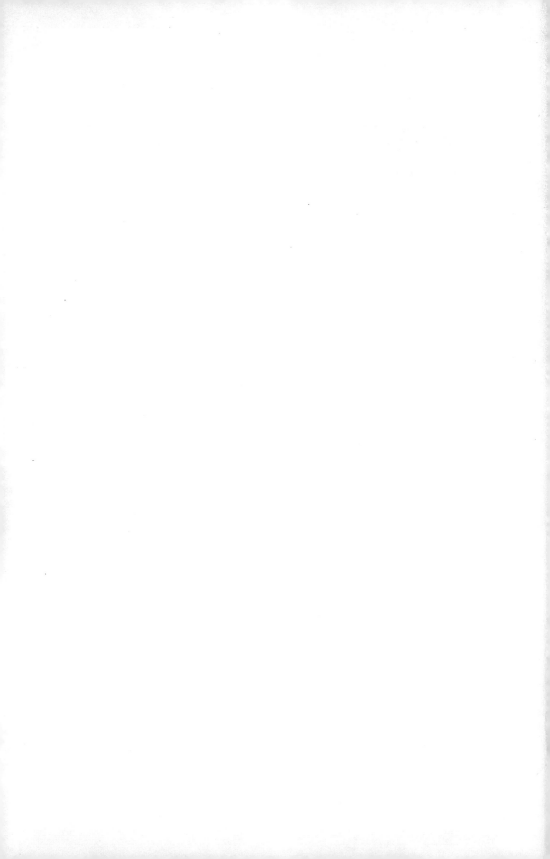

# ADVANCES IN
## Cardiac Surgery®

VOLUME 7

# ADVANCES IN
## Cardiac Surgery®

VOLUME 1 THROUGH 3 (OUT OF PRINT)

## VOLUME 4

# VOLUME 5

# VOLUME 6

# ADVANCES IN
# Cardiac Surgery®

VOLUME 7

**Editor-in-Chief**
**Robert B. Karp, M.D.**
Professor of Surgery, Chief of Cardiac Surgery, University of Chicago,
Pritzker School of Medicine, Chicago, Illinois

**Editorial Board**
**Hillel Laks, M.D.**
Professor and Chief, Division of Cardiothoracic Surgery, Director, Heart
Transplant Program, UCLA Medical Center, Los Angeles, California

**Andrew S. Wechsler, M.D.**
Stuart McGuire Professor and Chairman, Department of Surgery, Chief,
Division of Cardiothoracic Surgery, Professor of Physiology, Medical
College of Virginia, Virginia Commonwealth University, Richmond,
Virginia

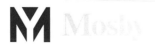

St. Louis  Baltimore  Boston  Carlsbad  Chicago  Naples  New York  Philadelphia  Portland
London  Madrid  Mexico City  Singapore  Sydney  Tokyo  Toronto  Wiesbaden

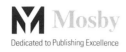

Dedicated to Publishing Excellence

A Times Mirror
Company

Vice President and Publisher, Continuity Publishing: Kenneth H. Killion
Director, Editorial Development: Gretchen C. Murphy
Developmental Editor: Lulu Danan
Acquisitions Editor: Jennifer Roche
Manager, Continuity–EDP: Maria Nevinger
Project Manager: Jill C. Waite
Assistant Project Supervisor: Sandra Rogers
Proofreading Supervisor: Barbara M. Kelly
Vice President, Professional Sales and Marketing: George M. Parker
Senior Marketing Manager: Eileen M. Lynch
Marketing Specialist: Lynn D. Stevenson

Printed in the United States of America
Composition by The Clarinda Company
Printing/binding by The Maple-Vail Book Manufacturing Group

Mosby–Year Book, Inc.
11830 Westline Industrial Drive
St. Louis, Missouri 63146

Editorial Office:
Mosby–Year Book, Inc.
200 North La Salle Street
Chicago, Illinois 60601

International Standard Serial Number: 0889-5074
International Standard Book Number: 0-8151-5098-9

# Contributors

**Vivekanand Allada, M.D.**
Division of Pediatric Cardiology, Department of Pediatrics, UCLA
Medical Center, Los Angeles

**Abbas Ardehali, M.D.**
Division of Cardiothoracic Surgery, Department of Surgery, UCLA
Medical Center, Los Angeles, California

**Robert H. Anderson, M.D.**
Professor, Department of Paediatrics, National Heart and Lung Institute,
London, England

**Elisabeth K. Beahm, M.D.**
Chief Resident, Section of Plastic and Reconstructive Surgery, University
of Chicago, Chicago, Illinois

**Arie Blitz, M.D.**
Division of Cardiothoracic Surgery, Department of Surgery, UCLA
School of Medicine, Los Angeles, California

**W. Morris Brown, M.D.**
Division of Cardiothoracic Surgery, Department of Surgery, Emory
University School of Medicine and Carlyle Fraser Heart Center,
Crawford Long Hospital of Emory University, Atlanta, Georgia

**Delos M. Cosgrove III, M.D.**
Cleveland Clinic Foundation, Department of Thoracic and
Cardiovascular Surgery, Cleveland, Ohio

**Joseph M. Craver, M.D.**
Division of Cardiothoracic Surgery, Department of Surgery, Emory
University School of Medicine and Carlyle Fraser Heart Center,
Crawford Long Hospital of Emory University, Atlanta, Georgia

**Charles D. Fraser, Jr., M.D.**
Cleveland Clinic Foundation, Department of Thoracic and
Cardiovascular Surgery, Cleveland, Ohio

**John Parker Gott, M.D.**
Division of Cardiothoracic Surgery, Department of Surgery, Emory
University School of Medicine and Carlyle Fraser Heart Center,
Crawford Long Hospital of Emory University, Atlanta, Georgia

### Lawrence J. Gottlieb, M.D.
Professor of Clinical Surgery, Section of Plastic and Reconstructive Surgery, University of Chicago, Chicago, Illinois

### Glenn P. Gravlee, M.D.
Professor and Chairman, Department of Anesthesiology, Allegheny Campus, Medical College of Pennsylvania and Hahnemann University, Pittsburgh, Pennsylvania

### Robert A. Guyton, M.D.
Division of Cardiothoracic Surgery, Department of Surgery, Emory University School of Medicine and Carlyle Fraser Heart Center, Crawford Long Hospital of Emory University, Atlanta, Georgia

### Robert B. Karp, M.D.
Professor of Surgery, Chief of Cardiac Surgery, University of Chicago, Pritzker School of Medicine, Chicago, Illinois

### Thomas J. Krizek, M.D.
Professor of Surgery, Vice-Chairman of the Department of Surgery and Chief of Plastic Surgery, University of South Florida, Tampa, Florida

### Hillel Laks, M.D.
Division of Cardiothoracic Surgery, Department of Surgery, UCLA School of Medicine, Los Angeles, California

### Jamshid Maddahi, M.D.
Division of Nuclear Medicine and Biophysics, Department of Molecular and Medical Pharmacology, UCLA School of Medicine, Los Angeles

### Albert Marchetti, M.D.
Medical Director, Physicians World Communications Group; Medical Director, Continuing Medical Education, Professional Services, Secaucus, New Jersey

### Michael Phelps, Ph.D.
Division of Nuclear Medicine and Biophysics, Department of Molecular and Medical Pharmacology, UCLA School of Medicine, Los Angeles, California

### Hideki Uemura, M.D.
Department of Cardiovascular Surgery, National Cardiovascular Center, Osaka, Japan; Department of Paediatrics, National Heart and Lung Institute, London, England

### Joe R. Utley, M.D.
Division of Cardiac Surgery, Spartanburg Regional Medical Center, Spartanburg, South Carolina; Clinical Professor of Surgery, Medical University of South Carolina, Charleston, South Carolina; University of South Carolina School of Medicine, Columbia, South Carolina

**Andrew S. Wechsler, M.D.**
Stuart McGuire Professor and Chairman, Department of Surgery, Medical College of Virginia, Virginia Commonwealth University, Richmond, Virginia

**Toshikatsu Yagihara, M.D.**
Department of Cardiovascular Surgery, National Cardiovascular Center, Osaka, Japan

# Contents

**Mosby Document Express**

Copies of the full text of journal articles referenced in this book are available by calling Mosby Document Express, toll-free, at 1-800-55-MOSBY.

With Mosby Document Express, you have convenient 24-hour-a-day access to literally every journal reference within this book. In fact, through Mosby Document Express, virtually any medical or scientific article can be located and delivered by FAX, overnight delivery service, international airmail, electronic transmission of bit-mapped images (via Internet), or regular mail. The average cost of a complete delivered copy of an article, including copyright clearance charges and first-class mail delivery, is $12.

For inquiries and pricing information, please call the toll-free number shown above.

# Cold and Warm Myocardial Protection Techniques

## Robert A. Guyton, M.D.

Division of Cardiothoracic Surgery, Department of Surgery, Emory
University School of Medicine and the Carlyle Fraser Heart Center,
Crawford Long Hospital of Emory University, Atlanta, Georgia

## John Parker Gott, M.D.

Division of Cardiothoracic Surgery, Department of Surgery, Emory
University School of Medicine and the Carlyle Fraser Heart Center,
Crawford Long Hospital of Emory University, Atlanta, Georgia

## W. Morris Brown, M.D.

Division of Cardiothoracic Surgery, Department of Surgery, Emory
University School of Medicine and the Carlyle Fraser Heart Center,
Crawford Long Hospital of Emory University, Atlanta, Georgia

## Joseph M. Craver, M.D.

Division of Cardiothoracic Surgery, Department of Surgery, Emory
University School of Medicine and the Carlyle Fraser Heart Center,
Crawford Long Hospital of Emory University, Atlanta, Georgia

M yocardial protection during cardiac operations has been a topic of investigation for some 40 years. Gradually systems of protection have been developed that have allowed the surgeon to operate on more and more difficult pathologic conditions. Cold myocardial protection depends on cessation of myocardial metabolism so that biochemical pathways, nutrient stores, and critical chemical compounds are "frozen" in a functional state. As the heart is rewarmed, this functional state is restored to a greater or lesser degree. Since literally freezing the heart (that is, taking the temperature down to 0° C or less), which could effect a near complete preservation of a particular biochemical state, actually causes cellular and subcellular damage, the heart must be protected with cold systems of protection at higher temperatures (temperatures of 2° C to 4° C have been used experimentally, but clinically temperatures of 10° C to 18° C are more common). At these higher clinical temperatures, metabolic processes continue. Systems of cardioplegia have therefore been developed that supply nutrients to the heart during the period of cold metabolic quiescence. Notably these have been systems of cold blood cardioplegia or oxygenated cold crystalloid cardioplegia.

Very recently, consideration has been given to a more complete system for supply of nutrients to the heart with the heart metabolically quiescent in a warm state. This system of continuous or nearly continuous warm blood cardioplegia depends on chemical cardiac arrest to decrease the heart's metabolic needs while supplying an abundance of nutrients and oxygen with continuous blood cardioplegia infusion. This discussion will describe the use of cold cardioplegia techniques and the introduction of warm blood cardioplegia techniques in our institution.

## COLD CARDIOPLEGIA TECHNIQUES

Cooling the heart has been a prominent part of myocardial protection since the beginning of heart surgery.[1] For every 10° C reduction in temperature in biological systems, the metabolic rate of chemical processes is reduced by a factor of approximately 2. The myocardium may be cooled by infusion of cold solutions into the coronary arteries (perfusion hypothermia), by systemic cooling on cardiopulmonary bypass, or by local cooling with iced saline slush, cold irrigation, or cooling pads around the heart. These techniques are all useful, but the most effective method of cooling the heart is perfusion hypothermia. Very cold solutions (as cold as 2° C) may be infused into the heart without damage to the myocardium. With crystalloid solutions, myocardial temperatures as cold as 4° C have been achieved with nearly complete subsequent recovery.[2] The optimal temperature for cold blood cardioplegia is probably a little higher (15° C to 20° C).

Perfusion hypothermia, particularly in the setting of coronary artery disease, is heterogeneous hypothermia. This heterogeneity in cooling leads to heterogeneous recovery of myocardial function.[3] Local topical hypothermic techniques (irrigation with a liquid or slush solution or cooling pads) leads to more uniform myocardial cooling and more uniform recovery after the ischemic interval.[4-6]

When cold cardioplegia techniques were initially introduced, there was considerable controversy as to whether cooling the heart by itself was sufficient and whether mechanical arrest was additive. In mid 1970s in Dr. Willard Daggett's laboratory a cold cardioplegia solution was infused into the heart with isolation of the left anterior descending (LAD) artery from the circumflex system.[7] With this technique a high-potassium solution could be infused into one of the two regions while a normokalemic solution could be infused into the second region. Sonomicrometer crystals were used to study regional contraction in the two regions. Each heart could be used as its own control, and regional shortening after the cardioplegic arrest interval could be compared in a single heart with a high-potassium solution in one region and a normokalemic solution in the other region. This study revealed a clear benefit of hyperkalemic cold cardiac arrest: there was an approximate three-fold difference in cardiac function in the high-potassium region as compared with the normokalemic region. *Chemical asystole is an important component of cold cardioplegic techniques.*

Although the general theory of cold myocardial protection techniques entails suspension of activity of biochemical processes, it must be understood that metabolic activity continues, even at low temperatures. Even more important may be the imbalance that occurs between metabolic processes as the heart is cooled. As the heart is cooled, the reaction rates of various chemical reactions decrease at various rates. High-energy reactions such as those involving the Na-K-adenosine triphosphatase (ATP) pump are particularly depressed as the myocardium is cooled, with a reduction in reaction rate of by a factor of 4 to 6 for every 10° C. This is in contrast to the general decrease in metabolic rate by a factor of only 2 per 10° C decrease. This leads to a gross imbalance of myocardial homeostatic mechanisms. Supplying oxygen and nutrients to a heart at 28° C will not necessarily result in the maintenance of normal cellular function. A cold heart is indeed a heart with a greatly reduced metabolic rate, but *metabolic activity continues and the metabolic processes are likely to be out of balance.*[8]

Because metabolic activity continues in a cold heart and because of the heterogeneity of myocardial cooling (and rewarming in the interval between cardioplegia infusions), the supply of nutrients and oxygen to the heart seemed like an attractive possibility for enhancement of cold cardioplegic techniques. The technique of cold blood cardioplegia was developed by Buckberg and colleagues in the late 1970s and early 1980s.[9] Although blood cardioplegia provides excellent buffering, nutrients for aerobic and anaerobic metabolic processes, and free radical scavenging agents, the presence of oxygen in the solution appears to be an important contributor to its efficacy.[10]

In the early 1980s as these cold blood cardioplegic techniques were being developed, we studied oxygenation of crystalloid cardioplegia as a technique that might enhance myocardial protection. Because the solubility of oxygen increases as a crystalloid solution is cooled, the oxygen content of a very cold crystalloid solution can be 3.5 mL $O_2$ per 100 mL of solution (vs. approximately 0.4 mL $O_2$ per 100 mL of solution in a nonoxygenated room-temperature solution). This technique of oxygenation of crystalloid solution was studied in an animal model that used a period of myocardial ischemia to increase the stress on the heart before cardioplegic arrest. This particular model used 30 minutes of ischemia in the circumflex region and 15 minutes of ischemia in the LAD region before cardioplegic arrest. In the circumflex region, recovery with oxygenated solution was approximately 50% of the preischemic regional shortening whereas recovery with the nonoxygenated solution was less than 10%. In the less ischemic LAD region, recovery was approximately 80% with the oxygenated solution and only approximately 50% with the nonoxygenated solution. Based on encouraging results in animal studies, oxygenation of clinical cardioplegic solutions was begun.[11] The benefits of oxygenation of crystalloid solutions have also been demonstrated by others.[12–14]

As oxygenated crystalloid cardioplegia was introduced into our clinical practice, levels of the MB fraction of creatine kinase (CKMB) were monitored as an indicator of myocardial damage. In uncomplicated coronary artery bypass patients there was no difference in CKMB release with unoxygenated vs. oxygenated cardioplegic solutions if the cross-clamp time was less than 29 minutes. If the cross-clamp time was extended ($\geq$29 minutes), CKMB release was approximately 2½ times as great in patients with unoxygenated cardioplegic solutions.[11] We became firmly convinced that oxygenation of the cardioplegic solution is an important component of cold crystalloid cardioplegic techniques. As discussed earlier, this represents a system for supply of the quiescent myocardium with oxygen and nutrients during the period of cold cardioplegic arrest.

Another important consideration in the use of cold cardioplegia techniques is that the cardioplegic solution should be nontoxic. A number of the solutions that have actually been used for clinical myocardial protection are cytotoxic.[15] This is especially true for solutions that are dissimilar from interstitial fluid. This becomes particularly important with infusion cardioplegic techniques in the presence of coronary artery disease. Some regions of the myocardium will receive as much as ten times the flow of cardioplegia per gram of muscle as compared with other regions. A number of additives have been proposed for cardioplegic solutions that in moderate doses are beneficial but in higher doses are harmful. It is important that the cardioplegic solution be beneficial to the heart whether it is administered in low or high doses.

The basic components of the optimal cold cardioplegic solution should be a physiologic crystalloid or blood solution buffered to a slightly alkaline pH that contains glucose at physiologic or slightly superphysiologic levels and potassium in sufficient quantity to lead to mechanical arrest. This solution should be oxygenated and should contain a small amount of calcium. This nontoxic solution should be delivered with pressure monitoring. In cases of tight proximal coronary stenoses, cardioplegia pressures as high as 150 mm Hg may be used to improve the distribution of cardioplegia beyond stenoses. Temperatures as low as 2° C have been used successfully in infusion cardioplegia.[2] Myocardial protection is optimal if both proximal and distal anastomoses are performed during a single cross-clamp interval. This leads to a slight prolongation of the operative procedure (as opposed to allowing the heart to begin to recover during performance of the proximal anastomoses), but in situations in which early and complete recovery is important, use of a single cross-clamp interval is critical.[16, 17] Retrograde cardioplegia has been successfully used as a technique for improving the homogeneity of cardioplegia delivery. It has been used in combination with antegrade cardioplegia delivery and also as a technique for maintenance of cardioplegia after antegrade induction. It should be noted that retrograde cardioplegia is also clearly heterogeneous, with relative hypoperfusion of the right ventricle and septum.[18, 19]

As the heart is reperfused after cold cardioplegic techniques, it is restored from a state of metabolic quiescence to a metabolically active state. The reperfusion milieu during this interval is quite important. Particularly after an ischemic insult, modification of the reperfusion conditions can reduce the subsequent loss of myocyte function and structure.[20–26] At least six factors seem to be important in reperfusion modification:

1.  Metabolic requirements should be reduced during reperfusion by maintaining chemical cardioplegic arrest during the first 10 minutes of reperfusion.[27]

2.  Aerobic metabolism should be maintained by adequate oxygen and substrate supply during early reperfusion. Glutamate may be a particularly important substrate for metabolism.[27–31]

3.  Hypercalcemia should be avoided in the first few minutes of reperfusion, and relative hypocalcemia may prevent some of the influx of calcium into cells and cellular organelles that occurs in the first 5 to 10 minutes of reperfusion.

4.  An alkalotic reperfusate seems superior to an acidotic reperfu-

sate because rapid restoration of intercellular pH seems to improve recovery of function.

5. Oxygen-derived free radicals appear to be damaging in early reperfusion.[32] Xanthine oxidase inhibitors, free radical scavengers, and mannitol may be effective in early reperfusion.[33, 34]

6. Leukocyte depletion appears to decrease damage consequent to reperfusion of ischemic myocardium by minimizing the local inflammatory response that occurs with reperfusion of ischemically damaged muscle.

The best condition for reperfusion is infusion of warm hyperkalemic blood into a vented heart that is empty and nonbeating such that all nutrients and oxygen may be used for metabolic restoration. This is a so-called warm reperfusion or "hot shot" technique. Even after the heart has been restored with this warm cardioplegia technique, a period of 20 to 30 minutes in a perfused, decompressed, beating state will allow more complete recovery of myocardial function. Proponents of cold oxygenated crystalloid techniques can achieve very nearly the same reperfusion conditions by infusion of a dose of crystalloid solution into the heart immediately before cross-clamp removal. This leads to a quiet (bradycardic) heart during the first few minutes after cross-clamp removal.[17]

Venting of the heart is an important consideration because ventricular distension greatly increases metabolic demands. This is particularly important immediately before and immediately after the cross-clamp interval. During cardioplegic arrest, moderate distension obviously does not lead to an increased demand. Passive decompression of the heart may be accomplished by manual massage, a stab wound in the pulmonary artery, elevation of the operating table, or amputation of the tip of the left atrial appendage. Passive decompression of the heart does not involve negative pressure within the heart, and therefore introduction of air into the cardiac chambers is minimal. If passive venting of the heart is not effective, active venting may be accomplished by placing a vent catheter into the left ventricle via the right superior pulmonary vein, by suction on the ascending aorta (using one of a variety of commercial cardioplegic infusion cannulas), or by suction on a vent in the pulmonary artery. All of these techniques may introduce air into the heart, so de-airing maneuvers must be carried out whenever active venting is used.[35, 36]

A particularly important consideration in cold cardioplegic techniques is that the technique be adapted to the pathology.[17] In the experimental laboratory we can develop myocardial protection techniques that are designed to protect normal hearts with nearly 100% success. When these same techniques are applied to pathologic conditions, however, complete protection is much less reliable. Myocardial protection must be flexible. Each patient should have the shortest and most gentle operation consistent with excellent protection. This allows for rapid recovery after the anesthetic interval. In addition to being flexible, myocardial protection should be standardized in a given institution. A standardized technique leads to fewer technical errors. We have used a flexible myocardial protection technique built on a standard foundation. The standard foundation is systemic cooling to 28° C, antegrade cold crystalloid oxygenated cardioplegia solution, infusion of additional cardioplegia via each vein graft, cross-clamping during distal anastomoses only, and passive ventricular decompression. This standard system is made flexible by opportunities for enhancement. These opportunities for enhancement include further systemic cooling, local irrigation of the pericardium with repeated doses of iced solution, proximal and distal anastomoses during a single cross-clamp interval, active venting of the heart, and reperfusate modification.

Implementation of our system of cardioplegic protection can be demonstrated by considering two scenarios. In a relatively healthy patient with a good left ventricle, the patient is not cooled on cardiopulmonary bypass. Local cooling of the pericardium is undertaken and cold oxygenated crystalloid cardioplegia solution is infused with distal anastomoses performed during the cross-clamp interval. The heart is rewarmed and metabolically restored while proximal anastomoses are performed with a side-biting clamp. This leads to a very short cardiopulmonary bypass time, a short operation, and a quick recovery for the patient. On the other hand, in a patient with hypertension (left ventricular hypertrophy), left main coronary artery stenosis, and ischemia in the operating room before cardiopulmonary bypass, different techniques are used. The patient is placed on cardiopulmonary bypass quickly, and myocardial perfusion pressure is maintained above 70 mm Hg until the cross-clamp is applied. β-blockade is given as soon as the patient is placed on cardiopulmonary bypass, and the heart is vented passively immediately after institution of bypass by amputation of the tip of the left atrial appendage. The patient is cooled to 25° C, and care is taken to maintain good perfusion pressure with an empty, beating heart until the cross-clamp is applied. This allows metabolic restoration of the heart. If the heart begins to dis-tend or if rhythm disturbances (such as ventricular fibrillation) occur, the heart is immediately arrested with cardioplegia infusion. High cardioplegia infusion pressure is used because of the patient's left main coronary artery stenosis. A vein is grafted to the ischemic area first, and distal and proximal anastomoses are performed during a single cross-clamp interval. Retrograde cardioplegia may or may not be used in addition to repeated antegrade infusion down the vein grafts. After all of the proximal anastomoses are completed, a final dose of cardioplegia solution is administered just before cross-clamp removal. The bradycardic empty beating heart is then rested on cardiopulmonary bypass for 20 to 30 minutes before ligation of the tip of the left atrial appendage and institution of myocardial work. When this flexible myocardial protection technique is used, oxygenated crystalloid methods have been very successful in situations of cardiogenic shock and poor left ventricular function.[37] The system requires intelligent application of the various enhancement methods as various pathologic situations are encountered.

## COLD BLOOD CARDIOPLEGIA TECHNIQUES

Cold blood cardioplegia techniques have been very successful clinically.[9, 38] The patient is generally cooled to 25° C to 28° C, and an infusion circuit mixes blood from the pump oxygenator with a crystalloid solution to achieve a cardioplegia solution with a hematocrit of 16 to 20, a potassium level of 20 to 25, an alkaline pH, and a low calcium level. Substrate enhancement with glutamate and aspartate is often used during the reperfusion. Many advocates of cold blood cardioplegia techniques advocate the use of warm induction of cardioplegia.[39] This warm induction is an infusion of warm cardioplegia solution at the beginning of the cross-clamp interval that is designed to replenish a metabolically depleted myocardium. Ordinarily this cardioplegia solution is delivered warm for 5 minutes with a pressure of 50 mm Hg. The temperature is then reduced to 5° C to 8° C by circulating the solution through a coil immersed in iced water or iced saline. Before removal of the aortic cross-clamp, warm blood cardioplegic solution is again infused to restore the metabolic state of the heart before cross-clamp removal. When the cross-clamp is removed, chemical cardioplegic arrest gradually terminates as the cardioplegic solution is flushed out of the heart and the normal metabolic state is restored.

In the mid 1980s we conducted a direct prospective comparison of cold oxygenated crystalloid techniques with cold blood techniques. In routine coronary bypass patients we found no superiority of cold blood techniques over crystalloid techniques.[40] In situations in which the patient comes to the operating room with acute ischemia or acute metabolic compromise, however, blood techniques seem clearly superior to crystalloid techniques.[38] Modification of reperfusion conditions with blood leads to a dramatic restoration of myocardial function and integrity.[20-22, 24, 41] Acute ischemia is a compelling indication for the use of blood cardioplegic techniques. As will be subsequently discussed, continuous warm blood techniques appear to offer some advantage over intermittent cold blood techniques for resuscitation of ischemic myocardium.[42, 43]

## WARM BLOOD CARDIOPLEGIA

Warm blood cardioplegic techniques were developed as an alternative to cold techniques. This development was prompted in part by the complexity of cold techniques when they were used for very complex pathologic conditions. Hypothermic techniques have problems.[8] Hypothermia leads to myocardial and systemic cellular edema. Hypothermia impairs enzyme function, particularly inhibiting calcium sequestration and removal. Hypothermia leads to decreased membrane stability and impairs ATP generation and utilization. It has detrimental effects on glucose utilization and oxygen uptake. Hypothermia leads to loss of local autoregulation and may thereby increase myocardial ischemia as the heart is cooled. It was suggested that warm cardioplegic techniques would prevent the problems of hypothermia and offer the advantage that optimal temperatures would be maintained for the maintenance of cellular homeostatic mechanisms. These pathways were obviously designed to function in balance at 37° C. Furthermore, with continuous aerobic cardioplegic techniques there is *no ischemic period* because there is continuous oxygen and nutrient delivery.

Warm blood cardioplegia was introduced as a clinical undertaking after a series of reports from Toronto claimed a remarkable improvement in myocardial protection.[44-49] Other early investigators supported these results.[50, 51] Continuous blood cardioplegia, including retrograde infusion via the coronary sinus, has been suggested since 1957 in the cardiac surgical literature.[52-55] The clinical results achieved in Toronto in high-risk patients with long cross-clamp times,[49] in patients with recent myocardial infarction,[48] and in patients with acute ischemic mitral insufficiency[44] suggested that the technique as clinically practiced in Toronto might offer unusual benefits, particularly in the resuscitation of metabolically reimpaired hearts.

The basic concept of warm blood cardioplegia is that an abundant supply of nutrients and oxygen is delivered relative to oxygen demand. Oxygen demand is reduced by asystole to approximately one tenth the demand of a beating, working heart. Oxygen and substrate are supplied at about one third to one half the rate of a beating, working heart. Since none of the oxygen and substrate must be used to supply external work, all of it is available for cellular homeostasis and replenishment of depleted cellular metabolites. Because this is a blood-based solution, free radical scavengers and buffers are abundantly available.

Antegrade continuous cardioplegic techniques as first used in Toronto were somewhat cumbersome because each graft had to be separately infused. The introduction of retrograde techniques[56] simplified the cardioplegia delivery system. The apparent advantages of this system led to widespread experimentation with this technique. A recent survey suggested that 10% of cardiac surgeons had used these techniques by 1992.[57]

## THE TECHNIQUE OF WARM BLOOD CARDIOPLEGIA

The original technique of warm blood cardioplegia proposed by the Toronto investigators consisted of a mixture of one part crystalloid solution to four parts of blood infused antegradely into the coronary vessels. The crystalloid solution was 1 L of 5% dextrose and water mixed with KCl, 100 mEq; magnesium, 18 mEq; trihydroxymetholaminomethane (THAM), 40 mL; and citrate-phosphate-dextrose (CPD), 20 mL. A 40-mEq KCl solution was used after induction of cardioplegia was completed. The initial high-potassium mixture had a final potassium concentration of 21 to 22 mEq/L, and the subsequent cardioplegia infusion had a potassium concentration of 11 mEq/L. Antegrade flow rates were approximately 200 mL/min, and retrograde flow rates were recommended to be at least 150 mL/min. Coronary sinus pressures were maintained at less than 40 mm Hg.[44-48]

Difficulty in visualization of the distal anastomosis was an immediately recognized problem with the antegrade technique. It was found that the cardioplegia solution could be safely turned off for several minutes to facilitate visualization. Experimental studies, however, suggested that there was some risk involved in interruption of warm blood cardioplegia, especially if one were attempting to resuscitate stunned myocardium.[58] Local control of the coronary artery with small vascular clamps or the use of a carbon dioxide gas blower to blow the blood away allowed visualization without cessation of the cardioplegia flow.[59]

Occasionally during continuous warm cardioplegia the heart began to beat during the cardioplegic infusion, and on occasion, reinfusion of a high-potassium solution failed to restore complete arrest. This seemed to especially be the case in patients with left main obstruction or in patients who otherwise might have high noncoronary collateral flow. When this situation was encountered, the heart was often cooled to increase the margin of safety for cardioplegic protection. Alternatively, a β-blocker was administered (such as esmolol, 50 or 100 mg as a bolus), which usually led to mechanical arrest.

A third concern with warm blood cardioplegia techniques relates to the nonhomogeneous delivery of retrograde cardioplegic solutions. The right ventricle and posterior septum seem particularly vulnerable to hypoperfusion. Colored microspheres and echocardiographic techniques have demonstrated inhomogeneous flow, with nutrient flow to the right ventricle less than 10% of the nutrient flow in the free wall of the left ventricle.[18, 19] Clinically, however, the right ventricle appears to be relatively well protected by retrograde warm blood techniques.[60] A recent study using echocardiographic visualization of sonicated microbubble-labeled albumin revealed great patient-to-patient variation in cardioplegia flow, with perplexingly decreased flow in some patients in the lateral wall. The same studies suggested that anaerobic lactate production with retrograde techniques was greater than with antegrade techniques.[61] The clinical problem with right ventricular protection has been minimal, perhaps suggesting that the techniques demonstrating inhomogeneity of flow might reflect flow only in capillary beds. Parts of the right ventricle may be supplied with oxygen and nutrients by flow through a venous plexus that bypasses the capillary beds. It is also possible that the atrium and right ventricle may receive some of their nutrient supply from intracavitary blood.

The fourth problem encountered with the early application of warm blood cardioplegia was systemic hyperkalemia and hyperglycemia. Serum glucose levels as high as 400 to 500 mg/dL were often observed, and infusion of insulin was necessary. This has led to modification of the crystalloid portion of the warm blood cardioplegia solution such that the glucose level is closer to physiologic levels. Hyperkalemia was an obvious consequence of the infusion of as much as 200 mEq of potassium into a patient during a 2-hour cross-clamp interval. This can be partially treated by diuretic administration at the beginning of the cross-clamp interval to facilitate potassium removal. Hyperkalemia after cross-clamp removal is not generally a problem *unless* mild aortic insufficiency is present. If this is the case, ineffective ventricular contraction after cross-clamp removal will lead to ventricular distension unless appropriate venting maneuvers are accomplished. To prevent systemic hyperkalemia, particularly with prolonged cross-clamp intervals, lower levels of potassium are often currently used.

Systemic normothermia during warm heart surgery leads to a concern that perfusion pressures remain adequate during the cardiopulmonary bypass interval. Pressures above 50 mm Hg are maintained, usually with the infusion of α-agonists. α-Agonists are more frequently necessary during warm heart surgery than during cold cardiopulmonary bypass.[62] Activation of cytokines or other vasodilators during warm cardiopulmonary bypass is likely responsible for this vasodilation.[63, 64]

The appropriate flow rate for cardioplegia infusion during warm blood surgery is a matter of considerable concern. The original suggestion that the cardioplegia flow rate should exceed 150 mL/min with a coronary sinus pressure less than 40 mm Hg remains appropriate, but when the heart is elevated for circumflex anastomoses, coronary sinus pressures are often elevated to 60, 70, or even 80 mm Hg with lower flow rates. Some investigators have advocated sampling of coronary arterial pH to ensure that adequate retrograde flow rates are achieved. If persistent acidosis exists, then poor recovery of the ventricle is likely.[65] Investigators in Toronto have found that a coronary sinus flow for retrograde warm cardioplegia of less than 100 mL/min leads to a high lactate production. A retrograde flow of 200 mL/min minimizes lactate production and prevents acidosis.[66] Higher flow rates seem particularly important in hypertrophied hearts. Flow rates as high as 250 or 300 mm Hg may be necessary in these situations to provide an adequate margin of safety for myocardial protection.

## LABORATORY EVALUATION OF RETROGRADE WARM BLOOD CARDIOPLEGIA

Warm blood cardioplegia was introduced in Toronto as a clinical experiment. Two studies conducted in our laboratories have demonstrated some of the benefits of warm blood cardioplegia. We have previously demonstrated that hypothermic techniques using using oxygenated crystalloid solutions could lead to nearly 100% recovery of metabolism and function if the heart was intact metabolically and functionally before cross-clamping. Continuous warm blood cardioplegia is most likely to be beneficial if the heart is *metabolically depleted* at the beginning of the cardioplegia interval. Because the heart remains normothermic and substrate is continuously supplied, mechanisms for cellular maintenance and repair should be well maintained to allow recovery of stunned myocardium during the cross-clamp interval. We designed two experimental studies: the first examined warm blood cardioplegia after global ischemia, and the second examined warm blood cardioplegia after an interval of regional ischemia.

The model of acute global myocardial ischemia evaluated in our laboratory consisted of a canine model with 15 minutes of global normothermic ischemia followed by a 1-hour cardioplegic arrest interval.[42] The warm blood technique (with antegrade induction followed by retrograde perfusion) was compared with the cold oxygenated crystalloid solution (our standard clinical technique at Emory University) and with the intermittent cold blood technique advocated by Buckberg (with warm terminal reperfusion and substrate enhancement with aspartate and glutamate). After cross-clamp removal, the heart was reperfused and end points determined 30, 60, and 90 minutes later. An ultrasonic crystal system was used to determine end-systolic pressure-volume relationships, diastolic function, and the preload recruitable stroke work relationship. The end-systolic pressure-volume relationship demonstrated no significant difference in systolic function among the three groups. A linearized stress-strain regression analysis revealed that the left ventricle was stiffer in both the cold blood and the cold crystalloid groups than in the warm blood group (Fig 1). The preload recruitable stroke work relationship demonstrated that overall left ventricular function was significantly better in the warm blood group than in either the cold blood group or the cold crystalloid group (see Fig 1). Notably, the electrocardiogram in the warm blood group appeared to return essentially to normal, whereas continued ST segment elevation was present in both of the cold groups (Fig 2). The salutary effect of cold blood cardioplegia in the resuscitation of ischemic or stunned myocardium has been well demonstrated.[20-22, 38, 40] This experimental study suggested that continuous warm cardioplegia delivered in a retrograde manner was at least as good as cold blood cardioplegia and certainly better than cold crystalloid cardioplegia in the resuscitation of ischemic myocardium. Since global ischemia is an unusual clinical situation, a second experimental model was designed to evaluate the potential benefit of continuous warm blood cardioplegia in the setting of regional myocardial ischemia.

A similar canine model was used, again with a triaxial sonomi-

# A Preload Recruitable Stroke Work

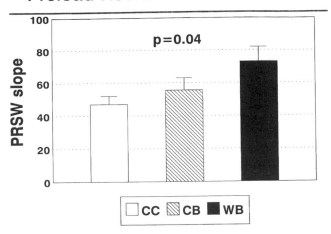

# B Stress-Strain Relationship

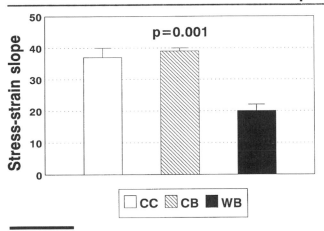

**FIGURE 1.**

In a model of global myocardial ischemia (15 minutes) followed by 1 hour of cardioplegic resuscitation, left ventricular function was better preserved by warm blood cardioplegia. Depicted is preload recruitable stroke work **(A)** in each of the three groups of animals 90 minutes after cardioplegic resuscitation. A linearized stress-stain relationship **(B)** showed that the cold crystalloid *(CC)* and cold blood *(CB)* groups had significantly stiffer left ventricles than the warm blood *(WB)* group. (From Guyton RA: Warm blood cardioplegia and normothermic cardiopulmonary bypass, in Mora C (ed): *Cardiopulmonary Bypass: Principles and Techniques of Extracorporeal Circulation.* New York, Springer-Verlag, 1995. Used by permission.)

## Electrocardiographic Data

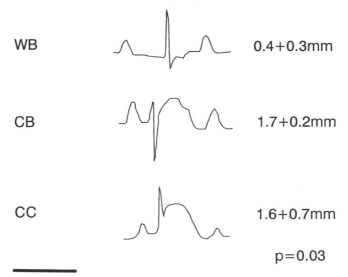

| | | |
|---|---|---|
| WB | | 0.4+0.3mm |
| CB | | 1.7+0.2mm |
| CC | | 1.6+0.7mm |
| | | p=0.03 |

**FIGURE 2.**

In a canine model of global ischemia (15 minutes) followed by 1 hour of cardioplegic resuscitation, the electrocardiograms consistently returned to almost normal in the warm blood *(WB)* group, whereas persistent ST elevation was observed in the cold blood *(CB)* and the cold crystalloid groups *(CC)*. Depicted are typical electrocardiograms and the average ST segment elevation for the groups. (From Guyton RA: Warm blood cardioplegia and normothermic cardiopulmonary bypass, in Mora C (ed): *Cardiopulmonary Bypass: Principles and Techniques of Extracorporeal Circulation.* New York, Springer-Verlag, 1995. Used by permission.)

crometer crystal system to precisely evaluate hemodynamic variables in a right heart bypass model of regional ischemia.[43] The LAD artery was occluded for 45 minutes followed by a 1-hour cardioplegic interval. The three cardioplegia groups were once again cold oxygenated crystalloid cardioplegia, cold intermittent blood cardioplegia with terminal warm reperfusion, and continuous warm blood cardioplegia delivered antegradely for induction and retrogradely for maintenance. Again, function was measured at 30, 60, and 90 minutes after reperfusion. Systolic function as measured by the maximum elastance relationship was superior in the warm blood group as compared with the cold blood group, which in turn was superior to the cold crystalloid group. Diastolic ventricular function was assessed by an active stress-strain relationship and revealed that both of the blood groups were superior to the cold crystalloid group. Overall left ventricular function was superior in the warm blood group as compared with the cold blood group, which in turn was superior to the cold crystalloid group (Fig 3). One of the more interesting aspects of this experimental study was that regional myocardial ATP levels in the LAD region were restored to normal levels after resuscitation of the ischemic region (that is, the LAD region levels were equivalent to the levels in the circumflex region). This occurred in the warm blood group but not in the cold crystalloid or in the cold blood group.

The very encouraging results with regard to resuscitation of ischemic myocardium with warm blood cardioplegia that were found in our canine models have not been fully supported in other

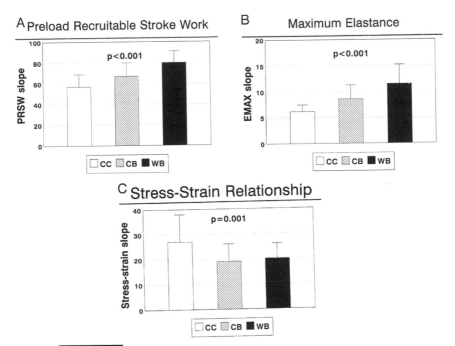

**FIGURE 3.**

In a model of regional myocardial ischemia (left anterior descending artery occluded for 45 minutes) followed by 1 hour of cardioplegic resuscitation, the warm blood *(WB)* group was significantly better than the cold blood *(CB)* or the oxygenated crystalloid *(CC)* groups with regard to preload recruitable stroke work **(A)** and maximum elastance **(B).** When the active stress-strain relationship **(C)** was examined, the slope of the stress-strain relationship revealed that the cold crystalloid group was stiffer than either the cold blood or the warm blood group. (From Guyton RA: Warm blood cardioplegia and normothermic cardiopulmonary bypass, in Mora C (ed): *Cardiopulmonary Bypass: Principles and Techniques of Extracorporeal Circulation.* New York, Springer-Verlag, 1995. Used by permission.)

laboratories. In a model of more severe global injury (45 minutes of normothermic ischemia), Kofski and colleagues from Buckberg's laboratory found that 30 minutes of cardioplegic reperfusion was damaging whereas 10 minutes of cardioplegic reperfusion led to prominent resuscitation. These authors believed that this represented an "overdose" of cardioplegia reperfusion.[67]

A second study conducted in Toronto in isolated blood-perfused pig hearts examined recovery of metabolites with nuclear magnetic resonance (NMR) spectroscopy. These pig hearts were subjected to a 20-minute period of normothermic ischemia before reperfusion with either normokalemic blood or cardioplegia solution. These investigators found a 30% to 40% loss of ATP levels in all groups that was *not* restored to normal with continuous cardioplegia infusion.[68] This result is consistent with other studies of stunned myocardium that indicate that the restoration of high-energy phosphate levels is a slow process requiring at least several days.

## CLINICAL EVALUATION OF WARM BLOOD CARDIOPLEGIA

Warm blood cardioplegia has been evaluated in two large prospective clinical trails. Martin and colleagues at Emory University compared continuous retrograde warm blood cardioplegia with the institutional standard oxygenated crystalloid cardioplegia.[69] This study was initiated after the warm blood technique had been used in over 300 patients and encouraging clinical results had been obtained.[70] In the warm blood group, systemic temperatures were maintained as close to 37° C as possible. This required active warming of the arterial blood if the systemic temperature fell below 36° C. Antegrade induction of cardioplegic arrest was accomplished and followed by continuous retrograde infusion of cardioplegic solution. Coronary sinus pressures were maintained below 40 mm Hg, which meant that coronary sinus infusion flow rates were often less than 150 mL/min (although an attempt was made to maintain a flow rate of 150 mL/min). High- and low-potassium solutions were used. Reinfusion of high-potassium solution was accomplished if the heart began to beat. In the cold oxygenated crystalloid group, cardioplegia was delivered with an initial antegrade dose of 1 L at a temperature of approximately 4° C. Additional cardioplegia solution was infused through the vein grafts as they were completed and/or through the coronary sinus, the aortic root, or a combination of these to maintain myocardial hypothermia. In both groups systemic flow was maintained at 2.2 L/min/m$^2$ with perfusion pressures of 50 to 70 mm Hg while the temperature was 32° C or greater. A lower systemic flow was used at colder temperatures as long as the systemic venous arterial saturation was above 90%. In the cold group, hypothermic systemic perfusion was accomplished at 25° C to 28° C.

Randomization was accomplished on 1,001 patients. Intraoperative and preoperative variables were similar. The aortic cross-clamp time was longer in the warm group (46 minutes vs. 40 minutes), and cardiopulmonary bypass times were similar, approximately 85 minutes in each group.

Mortality and morbidity results were remarkably similar for the two groups. The mortality rate was low (1.6% in the cold oxygenated crystalloid group and 1% in the warm blood group). The Q-wave infarction rate was 1% in each group, and the rate of intra-aortic balloon pump use was slightly under 2% in each group. The use of inotropic agents was 15% in each group. Myocardial function therefore seemed to be very well preserved in both groups, with a slight trend toward improved mortality in the warm cardioplegia group.

A very concerning difference was noted with regard to neurologic outcomes between the two groups during the course of the study. An acute perioperative cerebral vascular accident (a cerebral vascular accident occurring within 3 days of surgery and leading to a neurologic deficit at the time of discharge) occurred in 3.1% of the warm cardioplegia patients and in 1% of the patients in the cold crystalloid group (P < .02). An additional five patients in the warm blood cardioplegia group sustained a delayed cerebral vascular accident (more than 3 days after surgery but during hospitalization), and 1 patient in the cold crystalloid group had such a delayed cerebral vascular accident. Postoperative encephalopathy occurred in two patients in the warm group and one patient in the cold group. The difference in total neurologic events between the two groups was therefore 4.5% vs. 1.4% (P < .005). This adverse neurologic outcome led to a re-evaluation of this technique since warm blood cardioplegia, as practiced at Emory University, was clearly associated with an increased neurologic threat.[70]

A second large prospective trial of warm blood cardioplegia was conducted in Toronto to compare antegrade warm blood cardioplegia with antegrade cold blood cardioplegia.[71] The Toronto group actually used intermittent cardioplegia delivery in both groups, with the cardioplegia solution turned off during approximately 50% of the cross-clamp interval.[72] One thousand seven hundred thirty-two patients were randomized, with no differences found in preoperative variables. Mortality showed a nonsignificant trend toward superior results in the warm group (1.4% vs. 2.6%, P = .08). A significant difference was found between the two groups with regard to enzymatic detection of myocardial injury (12.6% in the warm group vs. 16.1% in the cold group, P < .05). A second significant difference was observed: fewer patients had a low-output syndrome postoperatively in the warm group (6% vs. 9.3%, P = .05). There was no difference in stroke between the two groups (1.6% for the warm group and 1.5% for the cold group).[71]

A comparison of the patients and particularly a comparison of the technical aspects of these two large prospective studies might reveal the important determinants of stoke in the Emory trial. The Toronto study excluded patients with internal carotid artery stenosis (>80%) or renal insufficiency. The Toronto series contained fewer females (16% vs. 25%) and fewer patients older than age 70 (approximately 16% vs. 30%). The Emory study included more patients who underwent reoperations (14% vs. 4%). Clearly, therefore, with fewer elderly patients, fewer reoperations, and fewer females, the Toronto series had a patient population with a lower susceptibility to stroke. Cardioplegia delivery in the Toronto trial was primarily antegrade (94% of the cases were exclusively antegrade) in both the cold blood and the warm blood groups. In the Emory trial all patients receiving warm blood cardioplegia received retrograde infusion. In both trials approximately half of the patients had proximal anastomoses performed with a partial-occlusion clamp. Cardiopulmonary bypass pressures and flow rates were similar in the two randomized series. Patients in the Emory series, however, were actively warmed to maintain systemic normothermia, whereas warm cardioplegia patients in the Toronto series had lower systemic temperatures that drifted to 30° C to 33° C. Both groups in the Toronto series were exposed to similar levels of hyperglycemia, whereas in the Emory series the warm blood group was significantly more hyperglycemic than the cold crystalloid group.

Multivariant analysis was carried out to determine the important predictors of stroke in the Emory group. Preoperative congestive heart failure was strongly associated with stoke, as was age and aortic cross-clamp time. The use of warm cardioplegia was an independent predictor of stroke (P = .026) in this multivariant analysis. The increased stroke rate in the warm blood group was confined primarily to elderly patients, with no difference in stroke rate in patients under the age of 60. This suggests an increased tendency toward stoke in the warm blood group, combined with an increased vulnerability in elderly patients (Fig 4).

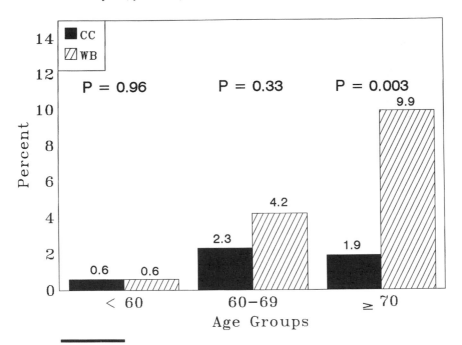

**FIGURE 4.**

A prospective randomized comparison of cold crystalloid cardioplegia and warm blood cardioplegia revealed an increased incidence of neurologic events in the warm blood (WB) patients vs. the cold crystalloid (CC) patients. This difference was primarily confined to the older patients, with no difference in the patients less than age 60 and a fivefold difference in the patients greater than age 70. (From Guyton RA, Mellitt R, Weintraub W: *J Card Surg*, in press. Used by permission.)

The etiology of stoke in the Emory patients appears to be an increased susceptibility to emboli because of the normothermic condition of the brain. Indeed, because the patients were often actively warmed to maintain normothermia, the brain in some patients may have been hyperthermic during critical portions of the operation. Cerebral emboli occur in all cardiac operations, particularly at the time of cannulation, during initiation of cardiopulmonary bypass, with cross-clamp removal, with partial-occlusion clamp placement, and with removal of the partial-occlusion clamp.[73] A correlation between these emboli and a subsequent neurologic adverse event has been observed.[73] The neurologic events found in the Emory study were focal, and one would presume that these were embolic in etiology. One must further presume that either there were more emboli in the warm group or that the cerebral susceptibility to emboli was greater.

The susceptibility of the brain to cerebral emboli is clearly greater during normothermia than during hypothermia. The metabolic rate of the brain is reduced during hypothermia. Cerebral venous desaturation has been observed in a much higher percentage of patients with normothermia than has been observed with hypothermic cardiopulmonary bypass.[74] Even a few degrees' temperature difference may lead to as much as a 50% reduction in brain metabolism.[75] Because systemic temperature in the Toronto series was allowed to fall, the brain was likely to be a few degrees below normothermia during aortic declamping, side-biting clamp placement, and side-biting clamp removal, those times that the bulk of cerebral emboli occur during coronary bypass operations.

Another possible ideology of increased cerebral susceptibility to emboli in the warm cardioplegia group in the Emory trial was an elevated glucose level. In the Toronto series a similar glucose load was infused in both the cold and the warm cardioplegia groups. In the Emory series the glucose level was markedly elevated in the warm group as compared with the cold group, with levels as high as 400 or 500 mg/dL in some patients. One might argue that the low stroke rate observed in Toronto despite the use of glucose in both groups suggests that glucose was not a causative factor. The Toronto series, however, contained fewer elderly patients, fewer females, and fewer repeat operations. All of these factors, especially age, would tend to decrease the overall stoke rate in such a series. Elevated glucose in the warm cardioplegia group in the Emory series may have been a causative factor in increased susceptibility to stoke, although multivariant analysis did not reveal glucose level to be an independent predictor of stroke.[76]

One of the authors involved in the Emory trial (J. M. C.) continued to use aerobic cardioplegia in his patients after the randomized trial. He reported his results in 379 subsequent patients treated with continuous retrograde aerobic cardioplegic techniques after August 1, 1992. Two changes were made in the technique. First, the glucose concentration in the crystalloid portion of the cardioplegia solution was changed to achieve nearly physiologic systemic glucose levels. Second, the systemic perfusion temperature (and the cardioplegia infusion temperature) was lowered to 30° C. The neurologic event rate in this group of patients was 1.8%, very similar to the 1.6% neurologic event rate in the cold crystalloid Emory group and the 1.6% stroke rate in the Toronto series. This dramatic change in stroke rate at Emory University with these two changes in cardioplegic technique suggests that mild hypothermia and prevention of hyperglycemia may be important protective considerations in the prevention of perioperative stroke when continuous warm cardioplegia is used.[77]

## TEPID MYOCARDIAL PROTECTION

As discussed in the previous section, there appears to be strong evidence that strict normothermia is detrimental with regard to cerebral susceptibility to injury during cardiopulmonary bypass. For this reason, clinical and laboratory investigations are currently in progress to evaluate mild hypothermia combined with continuous or nearly continuous cardioplegic techniques.

Our own studies of moderate hypothermia with continuous aerobic cardioplegia involved a canine model of regional myocardial ischemia followed by attempted resuscitation with cardioplegia. We were seeking to determine whether tepid cardioplegia could lead to myocardial resuscitation of ischemic myocardium that was as good, or almost as good, as warm cardioplegia. A 75-minute LAD artery occlusion was followed by a 60-minute cardioplegic arrest interval. Again, continuous blood cardioplegia was used with antegrade induction and retrograde maintenance. Cardioplegia was infused at 18° C, 28° C, or 37° C. Once again, hemodynamic end points were measured at 30, 60, and 90 minutes after reperfusion. Recovery of systolic ventricular function (maximum elastance) was not different among the three groups, although there was a trend toward slightly higher maximum elastance in the 18° C and 28° C groups as compared with the 37° C group. Global left ventricular performance (preload recruitable stroke work) was significantly better at 90 minutes after cross-clamp removal in the 18° C and 28° C groups as compared with the 37° C group. There was no difference in diastolic function among the three groups. There were only small differences among the groups in myocardial ATP levels, myocardial blood flow, and myocardial oxygen consumption. Oxygen consumption was significantly higher in the 37° C group after reperfusion than it was in the other two groups. This study suggests that moderate hypothermia for a 1-hour interval leads to resuscitation of ischemic myocardium that is as good as that achieved at 37° C.[78] If resuscitation of ischemic myocardium is as good with tepid cardioplegia as it is with normothermic cardioplegia *and* because the safety margin for delivery of oxygen and nutrients is much better with tepid cardioplegia than it is with normothermic cardioplegia (the lower temperature decreases the myocardial metabolic demand), then tepid cardioplegia should be superior to normothermic cardioplegia. It has the resuscitative advantages of normothermic cardioplegia, a greater safety margin for myocardium metabolism, and very likely, a greater safety margin for cerebral protection.

A second experimental study of cold and warm cardioplegia was recently reported in which miniature pigs received 30 minutes of ischemia before cardioplegic resuscitation. These data were interesting in that the pigs receiving warm continuous retrograde cardioplegia had limited right ventricular and left ventricular recovery. The piglets receiving cold (4° C) continuous retrograde cardioplegia had nearly 100% right ventricular and left ventricular functional recovery. When warm continuous retrograde cardioplegia was supplemented by *simultaneous* antegrade cardioplegic infusion, right ventricular and left ventricular recovery was complete. This suggests that either supplementation of cardioplegia delivery or lowering of oxygen demands by hypothermia may be beneficial.[79]

A clinical trial has been undertaken to compare cold (8° C), tepid (29° C), and warm (37° C) cardioplegia during both antegrade and retrograde techniques. This study revealed increased lactate production after *retrograde* cardioplegia with either tepid or warm cardioplegia. Left ventricular stroke work was greatest after warm or tepid *antegrade* cardioplegia. Combination cardioplegia, that is, antegrade *and* retrograde cardioplegia, led to more complete myocardial perfusion during arrest than either antegrade or retrograde cardioplegia alone. The results of this study suggests that *tepid combination* cardioplegia may be the superior mode of myocardial protection.[80]

## SUMMARY

Cold cardioplegia techniques are effective and reliable in most circumstances requiring cardiac operations. The cold oxygenated crystalloid technique used in our institution provides superior exposure of distal anastomoses and excellent protection *when the heart is metabolically intact at the onset of the cross-clamp interval.* If the heart is metabolically compromised before the cross-clamp interval, blood cardioplegia techniques appear to have a distinct advantage in the restoration of this compromised muscle. The clinical results from Toronto and our own experimental studies strongly suggest that continuous aerobic cardioplegic techniques are superior to intermittent cold blood techniques in the resuscitation of ischemic myocardium. As normothermic cardiopulmonary bypass and normothermic cardioplegic techniques were introduced in our institution, an increased rate of adverse neurologic outcomes was observed. Modification of the warm blood technique to allow mildly hypothermic, or *tepid*, cardiopulmonary bypass and cardioplegia temperatures along with prevention of hyperglycemia has reduced the stoke rate with continuous aerobic cardioplegia techniques to the level observed with our other methods of myocardial protection. Tepid continuous aerobic cardioplegia may be the superior technique available in 1994 for the resuscitation of ischemic or metabolically compromised myocardium during the performance of cardiac operations.

## REFERENCES

1. Shumway NE, Lower RR, Stoffer RC: Selective hypothermia of the heart in anoxic cardiac arrest. *Surg Gynecol Obstet* 109:750–754, 1959.
2. Johnson RE, Dorsey LM, Moye SJ, et al: Cardioplegia infusion: The safe limits of pressure and temperature. *J Thorac Cardiovasc Surg* 83:813–823, 1982.
3. Dorsey LM, Cogan TK, Silverstein JI, et al: Alterations in regional myocardial function after heterogeneous cardioplegia. *J Thorac Cardiovasc Surg* 86:70–79, 1983.
4. Dailey PO, Pfeffer TA, Wisniewski JB, et al: Clinical comparisons of methods of myocardial protection. *J Thorac Cardiovasc Surg* 93:324–336, 1987.
5. Landymore RW, Tice D, Trehan N, et al: Importance of topical hypothermia to ensure uniform myocardial cooling during coronary artery bypass. *J Thorac Cardiovasc Surg* 82:832–836, 1981.
6. Daggett WM, Jacocks A, Coleman WS, et al: Myocardial temperature mapping. Improved intraoperative myocardial preservation. *J Thorac Cardiovasc Surg* 82:883–888, 1981.
7. Guyton RA, Jacobs ML, Fowler BN, et al: Regional myocardial protection: Use of a new method to compare cold potassium cardioplegia with hypothermic coronary perfusion. *Circulation* 62(suppl 1):26–33, 1980.
8. Cameron DE, Gardner TJ: Principles of clinical hypothermia, in Chitwood WR (ed): *State of the Art Reviews. Myocardial Preservation: Clinical Applications.* Philadelphia, Hanley & Belfus, 1988, pp xiii–xxv.
9. Buckberg GD: A proposed "solution" to the cardioplegic controversy. *J Thorac Cardiovasc Surg* 77:809–815, 1979.
10. Vinten-Johansen J, Julian S, Yokoyama H, et al: Efficacy of myocardial protection with hypothermic blood cardioplegia depends on oxygen. *Ann Thorac Surg* 52:939–948, 1991.
11. Guyton RA, Dorsey LMA, Craver JM, et al: Improved myocardial recovery after cardioplegic arrest with an oxygenated crystalloid solution. *J Thorac Cardiovasc Surg* 89:877–887, 1985.

12. Oguma F, Imai S, Eguchi S: Role played by oxygen in myocardial protection with crystalloid cardioplegic solution. *Ann Thorac Surg* 42:172–179, 1986.
13. Hendren WG, O'Keefe DD, Geffin GA, et al: Maximal oxygenation of dilute blood cardioplegic solution. *Ann Thorac Surg* 44:48–52, 1987.
14. Ledingham SJM, Braimbridge MV, Hearse DJ: Improved myocardial protection by oxygenation of the St. Thomas' Hospital cardioplegic solutions. *J Thorac Cardiovasc Surg* 95:103–111, 1988.
15. Carpentier S, Murawsky M, Carpentier A: Cytotoxicity of cardioplegic solutions: Evaluation of tissue cultures. *Circulation* 64(suppl 2):90–95, 1981.
16. Yau TM, Weisel RD, Mickel DAG, et al: Optimal delivery of blood cardioplegia. *Circulation* 84(suppl 3):380–388, 1991.
17. Guyton RA: Cardiopulmonary bypass, cardioplegia, and central nervous system preservation: The surgeon's perspective, in *Cardiothoracic and Vascular Anesthesia Update*. Philadelphia, WB Saunders, 1990, pp 1–13.
18. Aronson S, Lee BK, Zaroff JG, et al: Myocardial distribution of cardioplegic solution after retrograde delivery in patients undergoing cardiac surgical procedures. *J Thorac Cardiovasc Surg* 105:214–221, 1993.
19. Huang AH, Sofola IO, Bufkin BL, et al: Retrograde cardioplegia distribution is not affected by coronary arterial venting or by coronary sinus pressure. *Ann Thorac Surg*, 58:1499–1504, 1994.
20. Vinten-Johansen J, Buckberg GD, Okamoto F, et al: Studies of controlled reperfusion after ischemia. V. Superiority of surgical versus medical reperfusion after regional ischemia. *J Thorac Cardiovasc Surg* 92:525–534, 1986.
21. Allen BS, Okamoto F, Buckberg GD, et al: Studies of controlled reperfusion after ischemia. XV. Immediate functional recovery after six hours of regional ischemia by careful control of conditions of reperfusion and composition of reperfusate. *J Thorac Cardiovasc Surg* 92:621–635, 1986.
22. Cheung EH, Arcidi JM Jr, Dorsey LMA, et al: Reperfusion of infarcting myocardium: Benefit of surgical reperfusion in a chronic model. *Ann Thorac Surg* 48:331–338, 1989.
23. Bottner RK, Wallace RB, Visner MS, et al: Reduction of myocardial infarction after emergency coronary artery bypass grafting for failed coronary angioplasty with use of a normothermic reperfusion cardioplegia protocol. *J Thorac Cardiovasc Surg* 101:1069–1075, 1991.
24. Julia PL, Buckberg GD, Acar C, et al: Studies of controlled reperfusion after ischemia. XXI. Reperfusate composition: Superiority of blood cardioplegia over crystalloid cardioplegia in limiting reperfusion damage. Importance of endogenous oxygen free radical scavengers in red blood cells. *J Thorac Cardiovasc Surg* 101:303–313, 1991.
25. Quillen J, Kofsky ER, Buckberg GD, et al: Studies of controlled reperfusion after ischemia. XXIII. Deleterious effects of simulated thrombolysis preceding simulated coronary artery bypass grafting with con-

trolled blood cardioplegic reperfusion. *J Thorac Cardiovasc Surg* 101:455–464, 1991.

26. Schaff HV, Goldman RA, Bulkley BH, et al: Hyperosmolar reperfusion following ischemic cardiac arrest. *Surgery* 89:141–150, 1981.

27. Lazar HL, Buckberg GD, Manganaro AM, et al: Myocardial energy replenishment and reversal of ischemic damage by substrate enhancement of secondary blood cardioplegia with amino acids during reperfusion. *J Thorac Cardiovasc Surg* 80:350–359, 1980.

28. Bolling SF, Bies LE, Bove EL, et al: Augmenting intracellular adenosine improves myocardial recovery. *J Thorac Cardiovasc Surg* 99:469–474, 1990.

29. Haas GS, DeBoer LWV, O'Keefe DD, et al: Reduction of postischemic myocardial dysfunction by substrate repletion during reperfusion. *Circulation* 70(suppl 1):65–74, 1984.

30. Svedjeholm R, Ekroth R, Joachimsson PO, et al: Myocardial uptake of amino acids and other substrates in relation to myocardial oxygen consumption four hours after cardiac operations. *J Thorac Cardiovasc Surg* 101:688–694, 1991.

31. Rosenkranz ER, Okamoto F, Buckberg GD, et al: Safety of prolonged aortic clamping with blood cardioplegia. II. Glutamate enrichment in energy-depleted hearts. *J Thorac Cardiovasc Surg* 88:402–410, 1984.

32. Ferreira R, Burgos M, Milei J, et al: Effect of supplementing cardioplegic solution with deferoxamine on reperfused human myocardium. *J Thorac Cardiovasc Surg* 100:708–714, 1990.

33. Chambers DJ, Braimbridge MV, Hearse DJ: Free radicals and cardioplegia: Allopurinol and oxypurinol reduce myocardial injury following ischemic arrest. *Ann Thorac Surg* 44:291–297, 1987.

34. Shlafer M, Kane PF, Kirsh MM: Superoxide dismutase plus catalase enhances the efficacy of hypothermic cardioplegia to protect the globally ischemic, reperfused heart. *J Thorac Cardiovasc Surg* 83:830–839, 1982.

35. Lucas SK, Gardner TJ, Elmer EB, et al: Comparison of the effects of left ventricular distention during cardioplegic-induced ischemic arrest and ventricular fibrillation. *Circulation* 62(suppl 1):42–49, 1980.

36. Little AG, Lin CY, Wernly JA, et al: Use of the pulmonary artery for left ventricular venting during cardiac operations. *J Thorac Cardiovasc Surg* 87:532–538, 1984.

37. Guyton RA, Arcidi JM Jr, Langford DA, et al: Emergency coronary bypass for cardiogenic shock. *Circulation* 76(suppl 5):22–27, 1987.

38. Barner HB: Blood cardioplegia: A review and comparison with crystalloid cardioplegia. *Ann Thorac Surg* 52:1354–1367, 1991.

39. Rosenkranz ER, Vinten-Johansen J, Buckberg GD, et al: Benefits of normothermic induction of blood cardioplegia in energy-depleted hearts with maintenance of arrest by multidose cold blood cardioplegic infusions. *J Thorac Cardiovasc Surg* 84:667–677, 1982.

40. Kauffman JN, Walker T, Lattouf O, et al: Reperfusion modification

with a simplified blood cardioplegia system compared with oxygenated crystalloid cardioplegia. *J Extracorporeal Technol* 23:26, 1992.

41. Rosenkranz ER, Okamoto F, Buckberg GD, et al: Safety of prolonged aortic clamping with blood cardioplegia. III. Aspartate enrichment of glutamate-blood cardioplegia in energy-depleted hearts after ischemic and reperfusion injury. *J Thorac Cardiovasc Surg* 91:428–435, 1986.

42. Brown WM, Jay JL, Gott JP, et al: Warm blood cardioplegia: Superior protection after acute myocardial ischemia. *Ann Thorac Surg* 55:32–42, 1993.

43. Horsley WS, Whitlark JD, Hall JD, et al: Revascularization for acute regional infarct: Superior protection with warm blood cardioplegia. *Ann Thorac Surg* 56:1228–1238, 1993.

44. Panos A, Cristakis GT, Lichtenstein SV, et al: Operation for acute post-infarction mitral insufficiency using continuous oxygenated blood cardioplegia. *Ann Thorac Surg* 48:816–819, 1989.

45. Lichtenstein SV, Salerno TA, Slutsky AS: Warm continuous cardioplegia versus intermittent hypothermic protection during cardiopulmonary bypass. Pro: Warm continuous cardioplegia is preferable to intermittent hypothermic cardioplegia for myocardial protection during cardiopulmonary bypass. *J Cardiothorac Anesth* 4:279–281, 1990.

46. Lichtenstein SV, Ashe KA, El-Daliti H, et al: Warm heart surgery. *J Thorac Cardiovasc Surg* 101:269–274, 1991.

47. Salerno TA, Houck JP, Barrozo CAM, et al: Retrograde continuous warm blood cardioplegia: A new concept in myocardial protection. *Ann Thorac Surg* 51:1023–1025, 1991.

48. Lichtenstein SV, Able JG, Salerno TA: Warm heart surgery and results of operation for recent myocardial infarction. *Ann Thorac Surg* 52:455–460, 1991.

49. Lichtenstein SV, Abel JG, Panos A, et al: Warm heart surgery: Experience with long cross-clamp times. *Ann Thorac Surg* 52:1009–1013, 1991.

50. Kay GL, Aoki A, Zubiate P, et al: Superior myocardial protection by normothermic aerobic arrest over ischemic arrest for high-risk patients. Presented at the 28th Annual Meeting of The Society of Thoracic Surgeons, Orlando Fla, Feb 3–5, 1992.

51. Vaughn CC, Opie JC, Florendo FT, et al: Warm blood cardioplegia. *Ann Thorac Surg* 55:1227–1232, 1993.

52. Gott VL, Gonzalez JL, Zuhdi MN, et al: Retrograde perfusion of the coronary sinus for direct vision aortic surgery. *Surg Gynecol Obstet* 104:319–328, 1957.

53. Gott VL, Gonzalez JL, Paneth M, et al: Cardiac retroperfusion with induced asystole for open-heart surgery upon the aortic valve or the coronary arteries. *Proc Soc Exp Biol Med* 94:689–692, 1957.

54. Bomfim V, Kaijser L, Bendz R, et al: Myocardial protection during aortic valve replacement: Cardiac metabolism and enzyme release follow-

ing continuous blood cardioplegia. *Scand J Thorac Cardiovasc Surg* 15:141–147, 1981.

55. Khuri SF, Warner KG, Josa M, et al: The superiority of continuous cold blood cardioplegia in the metabolic protection of the hypertrophied human heart. *J Thorac Cardiovasc Surg* 95:442–454, 1988.

56. Menasche P, Piwnica A: Cardioplegia by way of the coronary sinus for valvular and coronary surgery. *J Am Coll Cardiol* 18:628–636, 1991.

57. Robinson LA: Cardioplegic solutions in the 90's: Current perspective and national trends. Presented at Myocardial Preservation: Past Trends and Future Technology, Atlanta, Ga, Oct 16–17, 1992.

58. Matsuura H, Lazar HL, Yang XM, et al: Detrimental effects of interrupting warm blood cardioplegia during coronary revascularization. *J Thorac Cardiovasc Surg* 106:357–361, 1993.

59. Teoh KHT, Panos AI, Harmantas AA, et al: Optimal visualization of coronary artery anastomoses by gas jet. *Ann Thorac Surg* 52:564, 1991.

60. Lichtenstein SV, Abel JG, Slutsky A: Warm retrograde cardioplegia. Protection of the right ventricle in mitral valve operations. *J Thorac Cardiovasc Surg* 104:374–379, 1992.

61. Ikonomidis JS, Rao V, Weisel RD, et al: Inhomogeneous retrograde cardioplegia (abstract). *Circulation* 90(suppl 1):202, 1994.

62. Christakis GT, Koch JP, Deemar KA, et al: A randomized study of the systemic effects of warm heart surgery. *Ann Thorac Surg* 54:449–459, 1992.

63. Menasche P, Haydar S, Peynet J, et al: A potential mechanism of vasodilation after warm heart surgery. *J Thorac Cardiovasc Surg* 107:293–299, 1994.

64. Teoh KHT, Bradley CA, Gauldie J, et al: Steroid inhibition of cytokine mediated vasodilation after warm heart surgery (abstract). *Circulation* 90(suppl 1):202, 1994.

65. Gundry SR, Wang N, Bannon D, et al: Retrograde continuous warm blood cardioplegia: Maintenance of myocardial homeostasis in humans. *Ann Thorac Surg* 55:358–363, 1993.

66. Ikonomidis JS, Yau TM, Weisel RD, et al: Optimal flow rates for retrograde warm cardioplegia. *J Thorac Cardiovasc Surg* 107:510–529, 1994.

67. Kofsky ER, Julia PL, Buckberg GD: Overdose reperfusion of blood cardioplegic solution: A preventable cause of postischemic myocardial depression. *J Thorac Cardiovasc Surg* 101:275–283, 1991.

68. Deslauriers R, Kupryianov V, Ganghong T, et al: Magnetic resonance in cardiac surgery. Presented at Myocardial Preservation: Looking Toward the 21st Century, Chicago, Oct 7–8, 1994.

69. Martin TD, Craver JM, Gott JP, et al: Prospective, randomized trial of retrograde warm blood cardioplegia: Myocardial benefit and neurologic threat. *Ann Thorac Surg* 57:298–304, 1994.

70. Martin TD, Craver JM, Weintraub WS, et al: Warm blood versus cold

crystalloid cardioplegia: A case-matched comparison (abstract). Presented at the 65th Scientific Session of the American Heart Association, New Orleans, Nov 16–19, 1992.

71. Naylor DC, Lichtenstein SV, Fremes SE, et al: Randomised trial of normothermic versus hypothermic coronary bypass surgery. *Lancet* 343:559–563, 1994.

72. Fremes SE, Lichtenstein SV, Naylor CD, et al: Intermittent warm blood cardioplegia (abstract). *Circulation* 90(suppl 1):202, 1994.

73. Mills SA: Cerebral injury and cardiac operations. *Ann Thorac Surg* 56:586–591, 1993.

74. Cook DJ, Oliver WC, Orszulak TA, et al: A prospective, randomized comparison of cerebral venous oxygen saturation during normothermic and hypothermic cardiopulmonary bypass. *J Thorac Cardiovasc Surg* 107:1020–1029, 1994.

75. Schell RM, Kern FH, Greeley WJ, et al: Cerebral blood flow and metabolism during cardiopulmonary bypass. *Anesth Analg* 76:849–865, 1993.

76. Lanier WL: Glucose management during cardiopulmonary bypass: Cardiovascular and neurologic implications. *Anesth Analg* 72:423–427, 1991.

77. Craver JM, Weintraub WS, Guyton RA: Incidence of neurological events after coronary bypass surgery: Further observations from the Emory Warm Cardioplegia Trial. Presented at the 41st Annual Meeting of The Southern Thoracic Surgical Association, Marco Island, Fla, Nov 10–12, 1994.

78. Bufkin BL, Mellitt RJ, Gott JP, et al: Aerobic blood cardioplegia for revascularization of acute infarct: Effects of delivery temperature on myocardial protection. Presented at the 13th Annual Meeting of The Society of Thoracic Surgeons, New Orleans, Jan 31, 1994.

79. Ihnken K, Morita K, Buckberg GD, et al: Limited right ventricular recovery with warm continuous retrograde cardioplegia. Presented at Myocardial Preservation: Looking Toward the 21st Century, Chicago, Oct 7–8, 1994.

80. Ikonmidis JS, Hayashida N, Weisel RD, et al: Myocardial protection with different cardioplegic temperatures and directions. Presented at Myocardial Preservation: Looking Toward the 21st Century, Chicago, Oct 7–8, 1994.

# Pharmacologic Intervention for Acute Low Cardiac Output

**Albert Marchetti, M.D.**

Medical Director, Physicians World Communications Group; Medical Director, Continuing Medical Education, Professional Services, Secaucus, New Jersey

**Andrew S. Wechsler, M.D.**

Stuart McGuire Professor and Chairman, Department of Surgery, Medical College of Virginia, Virginia Common Wealth University, Richmond, Virginia

M ore than 750,000 cardiac surgeries are performed annually. As surgeries have become more sophisticated and widespread and the general population has aged, older and sicker patients undergo surgeries that were previously reserved for younger, healthier individuals. Older patients with more severe disease are generally more vulnerable to the physical challenge of surgery and the insult of ischemia/reperfusion injury. Separation from cardiopulmonary bypass becomes more difficult when ischemic arrest is superimposed on pre-existing cardiac dysfunction, especially in individuals with limited cardiac reserve. Consequently, the need is increased for blood product utilization, prolonged aortic cross-clamping and bypass time, and mechanical assistance with an intra-aortic balloon pump. In this setting, morbidity and mortality associated with the surgical procedure are also increased.

Perioperative and postoperative myocardial dysfunction is not limited to older patients with pre-existing disease, however. It can occur in any patient.[1] Preoperative assessment of risk factors for the development of cardiac dysfunction during and after surgery can be used to anticipate potential problems and necessary interventions. Numerous studies have indicated that poor preoperative systolic function, as indicated by a low ejection fraction, is predictive of the cardiac difficulty and acute low cardiac output that can exist or develop perioperatively and postoperatively.[2-4] Older age is another preoperative predictor, along with cardiac enlargement, female gender, and elevated left ventricular end-diastolic pressure.[5]

The overall operative risk for morbidity and mortality is further related to recent and past myocardial infarction, current or previous congestive heart failure, and a history of diabetes and hypertension. Intraoperative tachycardia, hypertension, hypotension, and ischemia may contribute to less than optimal outcomes.[6]

Irrespective of risk factors, some degree of systolic dysfunction will routinely exist in the hours to days after cardiac surgery, even after uncomplicated separation from cardiopulmonary bypass.[7–12] A slow return to pre-existing levels of function usually occurs after a nadir is reached about 4 hours after surgery.[7] Expecting such a recovery pattern will assist in the management of patients with acute and chronic low cardiac output,[1] some of whom may need pharmacologic or mechanical support if clinically significant dysfunction exists or develops and jeopardizes vital systemic perfusion. Other patients may initially require pharmacologic and/or mechanical assistance to separate from bypass. In addition to the previously mentioned preoperative factors that predict compromised left ventricular function in the postoperative period, longer duration of aortic cross-clamping and extended cardiopulmonary bypass time increase the likelihood that drug support will be needed.

An appraisal of the quality of cardiac function and the need for therapeutic intervention can often be made during surgery simply by observing the physical characteristics of the heart. A dilated, poorly contracting heart and a distended pulmonary artery are markers of poor cardiac performance. Low cardiac output in perioperative and postoperative periods can be identified more precisely by a low systemic blood pressure, small pulse pressure, and depressed dP/dt upstroke, especially as preload is increased. A decline in the oxygen saturation of mixed venous blood to 60% is cause for concern. Values below 50% discourage separation from bypass and signal the need for additional support.

## CHARACTERISTICS OF ACUTE HEART FAILURE

Acute heart failure or low cardiac output generally reflects systolic dysfunction of the left heart but can also have a diastolic component and involve the right heart.[13, 14] With left ventricular systolic dysfunction, stroke volume is reduced and end-systolic volume increases. Expanded end-systolic volume leads to an increase in end-diastolic volume and pressure, both of which shift the classic pressure-volume loop of systolic function to the right (Fig 1). During left ventricular diastolic dysfunction there is decreased chamber distensibility, and the diastolic pressure-volume curve shifts up and to the left (see Fig 1). Under these conditions, a small rise in volume causes a substantial rise in left filling pressure, and a higher diastolic pressure is required for any particular diastolic volume.

Although right heart failure may occur independently, it is generally secondary to left heart failure and the resultant increased pulmonary pressure, decreased left ventricular compliance, and ventricular interdependence.[13, 14] Right heart stroke volume, ejection fraction, and the rate of ejection decrease as the right ventricle dilates and fails. Right ventricular end-diastolic volume and pressure increase, along with mean right atrial pressure and mean systemic venous pressure. If failure is mild, these abnormalities may escape attention.

Vascular impedance and capacitance directly affect the ventricular performance of a damaged heart. Left ventricular preload depends on the capacitance of the pulmonary vasculature, right ventricular output, and left ventricular compliance. Right ventricular preload is affected by systemic venous capacitance and intra-

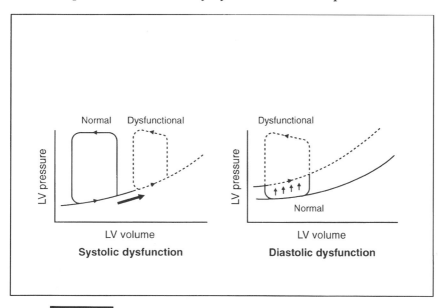

**FIGURE 1.**

Changes in left ventricular (LV) pressure and volume that accompany systolic and diastolic dysfunction.

vascular volume. Normal hearts augment systolic performance as preload increases (Starling effect), but failing hearts have an attenuated response to movements in preload. On the other hand, a heightened response generally accompanies a reduction in impedance because failing ventricles tolerate increased afterload so poorly.

## GOALS OF THERAPY

For patients with acute heart failure and acute low cardiac output, the primary goals of therapy are to improve cardiac performance and oxygen delivery to vital tissues. These goals can be achieved by (1) maintaining or restoring adequate intravascular volume, (2) reducing ventricular workload by decreasing systemic and pulmonary vascular impedance and ventricular preload, (3) improving myocardial contractility and diastolic relaxation, and (4) reducing or at least not increasing myocardial oxygen demand. Pharmacologic, catheter-based, or mechanical interventions that accomplish these objectives form the basis of treatment for the surgical patient with acute heart failure. Specific therapeutic goals and interventions (singular or multiple) must correlate with the particular needs of individual patients.

Based on the preoperative assessment of a patient for cardiac surgery, the following questions should be considered in anticipation of the need for aggressive intervention to support a failing heart during or after surgery: Is the patient at high risk for perioperative or postoperative cardiac dysfunction? Will the left and/or right heart be dysfunctional? Is the patient likely to experience difficulty separating from cardiopulmonary bypass? Will the patient need additional pharmacologic and/or mechanical support? Which pharmacologic agents offer the most benefit and match the specific needs of the patient? And finally, when should support begin? By anticipating need, a plan of action can be preconceived and initiated rapidly if necessary. Prophylactic pharmacologic support may also be indicated.

## CHOOSING THE BEST DRUG

Certainly, selection of appropriate pharmacologic intervention requires careful evaluation of the patient's clinical status before, during, and after surgery. In addition, basic physiologic and pharmacologic principles along with an appreciation of the benefits and limitations of current drug therapies must be kept in mind during the selection process. The choice of a specific agent depends on how that agent affects all the factors that determine cardiac output—heart rate, rhythm, ventricular preload and afterload, compliance, and contractility.

The selected drug should improve both systolic and diastolic function. Avoidance of tachycardia is important because an elevation in heart rate increases oxygen demand and subjects the heart to an increased risk of ischemia. Arrhythmias complicate weaning from cardiopulmonary bypass and in some cases necessitate pacing to maintain adequate cardiac output. Stabilization of blood pressure without producing hypertension or excessive vasodilation is critical because both can compromise a technically perfect cardiac operation. Bleeding from an anastomosis or an aortic suture line can result from severe hypertension, whereas hypotension may produce inadequate coronary perfusion with subsequent ischemia and further ventricular dysfunction. Severe hypotension also may jeopardize the perfusion of other vital organs, most notably the brain and kidney. Any drug selected should be easily titratable and rapid in its action and avoid abrupt shifts in blood pressure, tachycardia, and arrhythmias. Significant systemic toxicity (i.e., hematologic, renal, hepatic) further limits a drug's usefulness.[15]

## CURRENTLY AVAILABLE CARDIOTONIC AGENTS

### CALCIUM

Although the routine administration of calcium has occasionally been advocated to raise blood pressure and improve myocardial contraction after cardiopulmonary bypass,[16-19] the practice is generally discouraged.[20] In vitro studies have indicated that contractility can be enhanced in isolated myocytes by increasing the intracellular calcium concentration, but in vivo studies are not so convincing. Clinical evidence suggests that mean arterial blood pressure and blood levels of ionized calcium can be increased through the administration of calcium chloride, but the heart does not respond forcefully, and the cardiac index does not improve.[21, 22] Placebo-controlled studies have generated similar results.[23, 24] In addition, observations of cardiac surgery patients indicate that calcium concentrations, although slightly depressed during separation from bypass, quickly return to normal under the intrinsic control of parathyroid hormone.[25] Based on these and other studies, administration of calcium is unnecessary to normalize ionic concentrations after surgery unless the patient is hemodynamically unstable and severely hypocalcemic or severely hyperkalemic.[20, 24] In fact, calcium administration may actually be harmful and should be avoided when possible. It has the potential to increase calcium flux and contribute to perioperative stunning when given early during reperfusion. It has been associated with coronary artery spasm and ischemic injury[26]; moreover, it has been implicated in the development of postoperative pancreatitis following large-dose administration during surgery[19] and has thwarted the therapeutic response to β-adrenergic agonists such as epinephrine and dobutamine.[27] Interestingly, phosphodiesterase (PDE) inhibitors circumvent the dulling effect that calcium may have on other drugs with inotropic qualities.

## VASODILATORS

Afterload reduction is an important consideration and objective in the treatment of patients with heart failure or acute low cardiac output. To this end, vasodilators are particularly useful because they have the ability to expand the vascular bed through venous pooling and a reduction in arterial impedance.[28] The two vasodilators most often used in cardiac surgery during separation from cardiopulmonary bypass are nitroglycerin and nitroprusside.

Both of these agents are converted to a pharmacologically active metabolite, nitric oxide, which in turn activates guanylate cyclase and leads to the intracellular synthesis of cyclic guanosine monophosphate (cGMP) in smooth muscle and other tissues.[29-32] The precise role of cGMP in vasodilation is still obscure but appears to be related to the activation of cGMP-dependent protein kinase, which modulates the phosphorylation of various proteins in smooth muscle and leads to dephosphorylation of the myosin light chain. Muscular contraction is subsequently impaired and a state of relaxation is maintained. Physiologically, nitric oxide has the same effect on vascular smooth muscle tone as endothelial-derived relaxing factor, which causes some investigators to speculate that the two may actually be one and the same.[30-34]

Vasodilators help to unload the heart and favorably affect left ventricular function. With just modest afterload reduction of a markedly dilated left ventricle, a significant increase in ejection fraction can be achieved. Reduction of end-diastolic volume may not be as dramatic, but a decrease in filling pressure is frequently realized. Atrial pressures can also be reduced.

The impact on stroke volume depends largely on changes in left ventricular end-diastolic volume. With venodilation, end-diastolic volume and stroke volume are reduced. With arterial dilation, stroke volume is improved because flow is augmented.

Thus, venodilators affect congestive phenomena whereas arterial dilators facilitate cardiac output.[35]

## Nitroglycerin

Nitroglycerin is predominantly a venodilator,[36] but its effects on venous and arterial vessels are highly variable and patient dependent.[37] Venodilation leads to a reduction in left and right ventricular end-diastolic pressures. To a lesser extent, arteriolar dilation results in a decrease in systemic arterial pressure.[38] The notable venous dilation and mild arteriolar dilation that generally follow nitroglycerin administration reduce stroke volume. A summation of these hemodynamic effects can be visualized as compression and a left shift of the pressure-volume loop depicting left ventricular function during systolic failure (Fig 2).

The effect of nitroglycerin on cardiac output will vary with its impact on arteries and veins. Cardiac output will decline as a result of venodilation in patients with heart failure and normal filling pressures. On the other hand, cardiac output will increase modestly in patients with heart failure associated with elevated pulmonary capillary pressure and high filling pressures. These patients realize a decrease in congestive symptoms because nitroglycerin produces pulmonary and systemic vasodilation that reduces ventricular filling pressure and improves cardiac output. Increased cardiac performance will be upheld as long as an adequate filling pressure is maintained.

The most significant adverse effect of nitroglycerin is the excessive hypotension that results from vasodilation, venous pooling, decreased cardiac output, and reflex tachycardia.[36] No specific antagonist is known for nitroglycerin's vasodilator effects, so expansion of central fluid volume may be required to overcome the venodilation and arterial hypovolemia that accompany excessive dilation. The tachycardia that occasionally follows nitroglycerin administration is secondary to decreased cardiac output and can be detrimental if it increases the oxygen demand of a heart that is poorly perfused and already ischemic. Tolerance to the drug may develop rapidly and attenuate its effect on different parts of the circulation.[39]

## Nitroprusside

Nitroprusside is a vasodilator that affects the arteriolar and venous circulation in a more balanced way than nitroglycerin does. Arteriolar dilation reduces systemic vascular resistance, whereas venodilation concomitantly expands capacitance. Consequently,

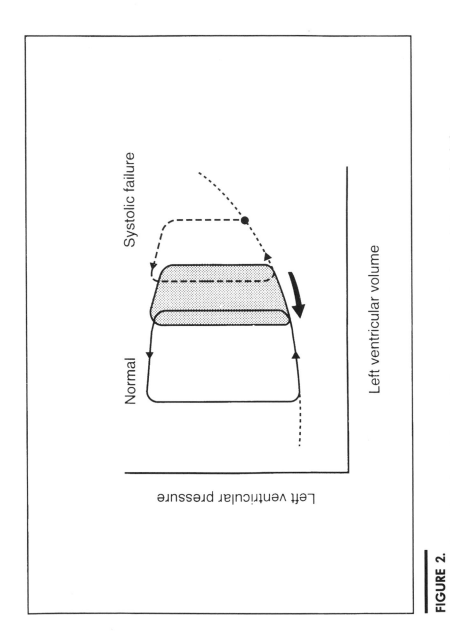

**FIGURE 2.**

The effect of nitroglycerin on left ventricular pressure and volume during systolic failure.

afterload and preload diminish while stroke volume is maintained and cardiac output is increased. These effects on hemodynamics and cardiac function shift the pressure-volume loop that is representative of systolic failure to the left while expanding the horizontal (stroke volume) component (Fig 3).

In addition to the general vasodilation produced by nitroprusside, cerebral blood flow is selectively enhanced[40] and pulmonary vasculature is dilated,[41] but the renal and splanchnic circulation may be critically compromised. Because of a coronary "steal" phenomenon, myocardial ischemia may worsen after nitroprusside administration,[42] so use immediately after the onset of acute myocardial infarction is discouraged. The benefit of nitroprusside in this latter setting may reside in late intervention when persistently depressed cardiac performance can be improved through preload and afterload reduction.[43, 44]

Nitroprusside is used to increase cardiac output and reduce pulmonary congestion during the short-term management of unstable patients with acute left ventricular failure. Additional uses include control of arterial pressure in aortic dissection (with a β-adrenergic antagonist), reduction in blood pressure during a hypertensive crisis, improvement in left ventricular performance after acute myocardial infarction or during severe congestive failure, and production of controlled hypotension during surgery.[28]

As with nitroglycerin, excessive vasodilation and severe hypotension are the most significant adverse effects that can accompany nitroprusside use. Because of the potential for hypotension and secondary ischemia of vital tissues and organs, close monitoring of blood pressure and the infusion rate is essential. Thiocyanate toxicity is also associated with nitroprusside use and can occur if nitroprusside is infused at a rate in excess of 5 μg/kg/min.[45]

## SYMPATHOMIMETICS

The catecholamines (epinephrine, norepinephrine, and dopamine) and their derivatives (dobutamine and isoproterenol) are used to support cardiac output before, during, and after surgery. The specific physiologic action of each of these drugs (Fig 4) relates to their relative specificity for α- or β-adrenergic receptors.[46]

$\alpha_1$-Adrenergic receptors are found in vascular smooth muscle and myocardium where their stimulation respectively causes vasoconstriction and a slight increase in myocardial contractility (positive inotropy) coupled with a decrease in heart rate (negative chronotropy). $\alpha_2$-Adrenergic receptors, also located in vascular smooth muscle, produce selective regional vasoconstriction when

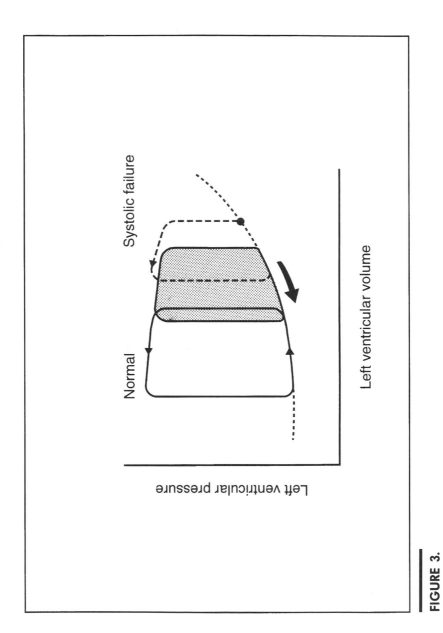

**FIGURE 3.**
The effect of nitroprusside on left ventricular pressure and volume during systolic failure.

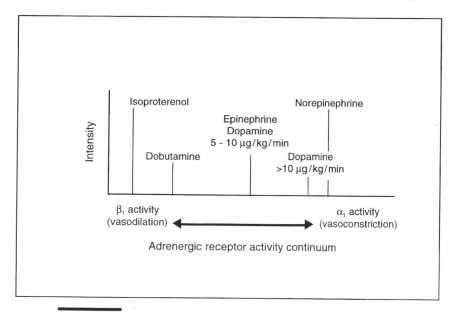

**FIGURE 4.**

The pharmacologic effect of sympathomimetic agents relates to their selective affinity for α and β receptors. (From McEvoy GK (ed): *AHFS Drug Information*, Bethesda, Md, American Society of Health-System Pharmacists, 1992. Used by permission.)

stimulated.[47] Other widespread effects of $\alpha_2$ receptor activation are mediated through the central nervous system.

Stimulation of $\beta_1$ receptors, which are located in the myocardium, produces positive inotropic, chronotropic, and dromotropic effects on the heart. The $\beta_2$ receptors that are found in smooth muscle cause vasodilation, whereas those found in the sinoatrial node increase the heart rate when stimulated.

The inotropic effect of these drugs is probably mediated through the increased delivery of ionic calcium and/or the heightened affinity of the contractile apparatus for calcium.[48] Activation of $\beta_1$ receptors increases the amount of cyclic adenosine monophosphate (cAMP) in myocytes, which in turn initiates cAMP-dependent protein kinase (Fig 5). These actions modify the sarcoplasmic reticulum and increase calcium ion flux and myofibril sensitivity to the ion.[49]

Contraction begins when calcium is released from the terminal cisterns of the sarcoplasmic reticulum. Subsequent binding of ionic calcium to troponin C, weakening of the troponin I–actin connection, movement of tropomyosin, and exposure of myosin

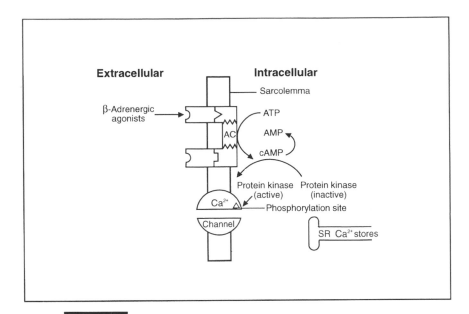

**FIGURE 5.**

Sympathomimetic drugs exert an inotropic effect on the heart by stimulating cyclic adenosine monophosphate (cAMP) production. SR = sarcoplasmic reticulum; ATP = adenosine triphosphate. (From Colucci WS, Wright RF, Braunwald E: *N Engl J Med* 314:290–299. Used by permission.)

binding sites allow actin and myosin to link and the myocytes to contract. Shortly after being released from the sarcoplasmic reticulum, however, calcium is actively reaccumulated and restored to the terminal cisterns. As the concentration of calcium ion diminishes outside of the reticulum, the interaction between actin and myosin ends and the myocyte relaxes.[50]

The molecular mechanism for vascular smooth muscle contraction via $\alpha_1$ receptor stimulation is through the increased formation of inositol-1,4,5-triphosphate ($IP_3$) and diacylglycerol (DAG), which results in increased cytosolic calcium primarily because of receptor-stimulated increases in phospholipase C.

The relaxation of vascular smooth muscle from $\beta_2$ stimulation is due to the activation of adenyl cyclase, which subsequently activates cAMP, which then activates protein kinase A.

## Dopamine

Dopamine is a naturally occurring catecholamine and a precursor to norepinephrine. Its positive inotropic and chronotropic effects on the heart are the result of direct adrenergic stimulation and also the release of norepinephrine from sympathetic nerve endings. At very low infusion rates, 0.5 to 2 µg/kg/min, dopamine causes vasodilation and occasionally hypotension through agonistic action on dopamine receptors, which are distinct from α- and β-adrenergic receptors[33]. The renal, mesenteric, coronary, and cerebral vasculatures are preferentially affected. By improving renal blood flow, urine output is enhanced. At moderate infusion rates, 5 to 10 µg/kg/min, the drug affects both $\alpha_1$ and $\beta_1$ receptors and thus improves cardiac contractility and increases the heart rate.[35] Hence dopamine can increase cardiac output with minimal effects on stroke volume. At infusion rates above 10 µg/kg/min, $\alpha_1$ activity occurs and produces vasoconstriction and a rise in blood pressure. The vasopressor properties of dopamine are sometimes helpful to maintain coronary perfusion pressure, but the drug has been shown to heighten the potential for infarction of ischemic tissues by reducing myocardial blood flow.[51, 52] As with other catecholamines, at higher infusion rates dopamine frequently causes tachycardia and arrhythmias.[53–55]

### Epinephrine

Epinephrine is another naturally occurring catecholamine that activates adrenergic receptors and imitates all of the actions of the sympathetic nervous system (PDR), including all of those outside the cardiovascular system. Its effects on the heart and blood vessels are similar to those of dopamine administered at moderate infusion rates. Of all of the catecholamines, it is the most potent α-adrenergic agonist. At routine doses, however, its most prominent actions are on the β-receptors of the heart and peripheral vasculature. At high doses, α-adrenergic effects predominate. Intravenous injection produces a rapid rise in blood pressure (mainly systolic), a direct stimulation of cardiac muscle that increases the strength of ventricular contraction, a rise in heart rate, and a constriction of the arterioles in the skin, mucosa, and splanchnic areas of circulation.

A research study comparing the hemodynamic effects of epinephrine and dobutamine has demonstrated that epinephrine increases the heart rate by less than 5% and dobutamine increases the heart rate by almost 20% when both drugs are administered at doses that increased stroke volume by 10% to 15%.[56] Furthermore, epinephrine appears to produce less tachycardia than dopamine or dobutamine at comparable doses. Tachycardia, hypertension, and visceral artery vasoconstriction can be problematic, however, when epinephrine is infused at a rapid rate or administered in high doses.

## Norepinephrine

Norepinephrine is another powerful stimulator of both $\alpha$- and $\beta$-adrenergic receptors. The drug has particularly strong $\alpha_1$ activity that leads to vasoconstriction of both the arterial and venous beds and, subsequently, elevated blood pressure. It also has powerful $\beta_1$ activity that enhances myocardial contractility and produces a positive inotropic effect. Although contractility is improved, end-systolic and end-diastolic pressures are increased because of greater arterial impedance secondary to the drug's vasoconstrictive properties. Venous return to the heart is also increased. Thus, the pressure-volume loop representative of systolic failure shifts to the right in response to norepinephrine (Fig 6). Significant adverse effects include hypertension and secondary reflex bradycardia.

## Dobutamine

Dobutamine, a catecholamine derivative, is a more recent addition to the list of clinically available adrenergic agonists. Although it stimulates both $\alpha$ and $\beta$ receptors, its primary effect is exerted through the $\beta_1$ receptor.[35, 57, 58] Cardiac contractility is enhanced and a positive inotropic response is noted quickly after intravenous administration. The heart rate also rises, but to a lesser extent than expected.[59]

Dobutamine's effect on the peripheral vasculature is more complicated. A combination of $\beta$ and $\alpha_1$ stimulation overrides any selective effect on individual receptors; consequently, no significant change in status occurs—impedance and arterial pressure remain relatively constant. Under these conditions, even though cardiac output is improved by augmenting contractility and increasing the heart rate, only a modest increase in stroke volume is realized.[52, 60, 61] The summation of all these hemodynamic effects is a left shift of the pressure-volume loop depicting left ventricular function during systolic failure (Fig 7).

In an attempt to identify the benefits and limitations associated with the clinical use of dobutamine in acute heart failure or exacerbated chronic heart failure, numerous comparisons have been made between it and other cardiotonic drugs. Unlike dopamine, dobutamine does not cause the release of endogenous norepinephrine and therefore does not evoke an additional indirect response through another agent.[33] It has a greater positive effect on cardiac output than dopamine does but also produces more tachycardia and less improvement in stroke volume.[51, 53] Although both drugs increase myocardial oxygen consumption in patients paced at 110

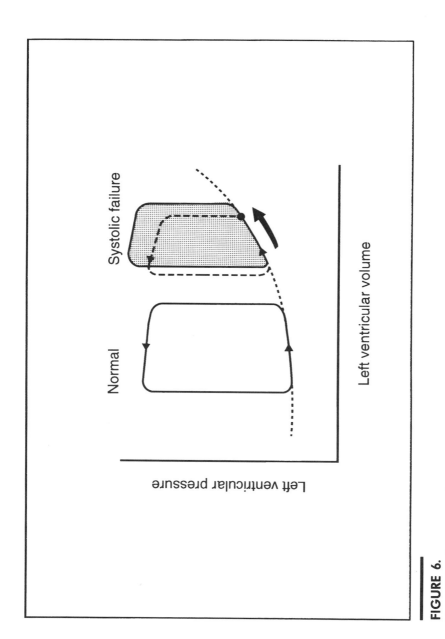

**FIGURE 6.**
The effect of norepinephrine on left ventricular pressure and volume during systolic failure.

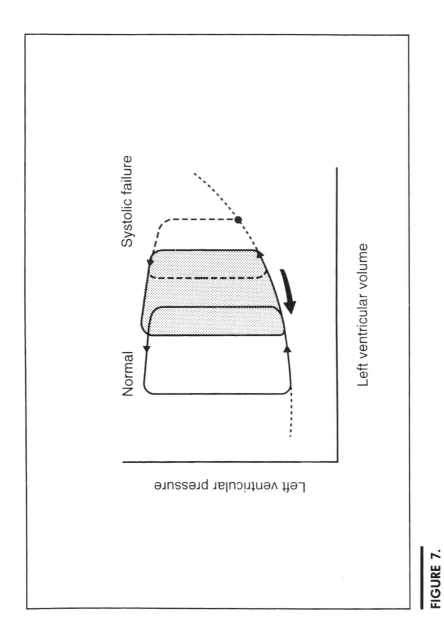

**FIGURE 7.**
The effect of dobutamine on left ventricular pressure and volume during systolic failure.

beats per minute, dobutamine facilitates more coronary artery blood flow.[52] With enhanced myocardial blood flow, dobutamine facilitates oxygen delivery and has a more favorable metabolic effect on ischemic myocardium than dopamine does.[54, 55, 60] The benefit of enhanced coronary perfusion, however, may be limited by the tachycardia caused by the drug.[55, 62] Dobutamine has been shown to induce greater tachycardia than epinephrine at doses that produce comparable increases in stroke volume.[52] Moreover, high doses of dobutamine may cause not only tachycardia but also arrhythmias, common problems associated with patients who are already predisposed to abnormal cardiac rates and rhythms.

### Isoproterenol
Structurally related to epinephrine, isoproterenol is a synthetic sympathomimetic amine that acts almost exclusively on the $\beta$-adrenergic receptor.[33] $\beta_1$-Adrenergic activity causes a marked increase in myocardial contractility and an increase in heart rate, whereas $\beta_2$ activity provokes peripheral vasodilation that helps to diminish afterload and preload. Although cardiac output increases following isoproterenol infusion, the stroke volume remains essentially unchanged. Systemic and pulmonary vascular resistance is decreased and coronary and renal blood flow is increased. Mean arterial blood pressure may decline or remain unchanged. The overall hemodynamic effect of these actions produces a left shift in the pressure-volume loop that depicts left ventricular systolic failure (Fig 8).

The usefulness of isoproterenol may be compromised by its propensity to provoke tachycardia, arrhythmia, and hypotension. Peripheral vasodilation may reduce diastolic blood pressure and limit coronary flow at a time when myocardial oxygen requirements are increasing as a consequence of enhanced inotropic effect.

## PHOSPHODIESTERASE INHIBITORS
Phosphodiesterase (PDE) inhibitors represent a relatively new class of drugs used in the short-term treatment of patients with moderate to severe acute heart failure, worsening chronic heart failure, and low cardiac output states. Currently, two intravenous PDE inhibitors are clinically available: amrinone and milrinone. Although similar to their pharmacologic and hemodynamic action, milrinone is 15 times more potent than amrinone milligram for milligram and has a shorter mean terminal elimination half-life and a shorter duration of action. Their mode of action is the same, however. Both

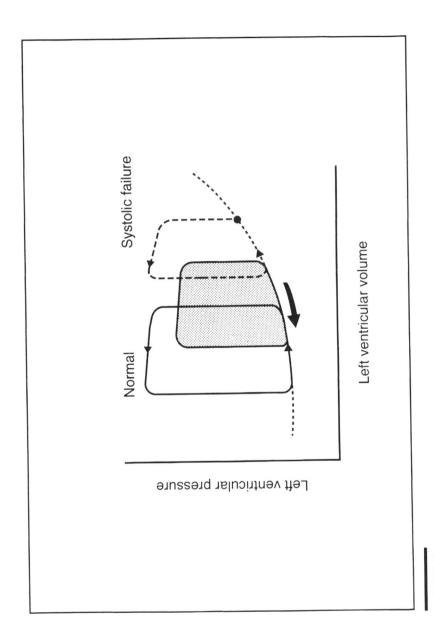

**FIGURE 8.**
The effect of isoproterenol on left ventricular pressure and volume during systolic failure.

drugs inhibit peak PDE III isoenzyme, which predominates in myocardium, vascular smooth muscle, and platelets. The isoenzyme is specific for cAMP and has no effect on cGMP or calmodium. Phosphodiesterase III inhibition results in increased levels of cAMP (Fig 9).

As previously discussed, the influx of ionic calcium from the extracellular fluid during each depolarization stimulates the sarcoplasmic reticulum to release stored calcium, which subsequently initiates myocellular contraction. As calcium is actively reaccumulated and restored to the terminal cisterns, the myocyte relaxes. The calcium current is cAMP dependent. In heart failure, less calcium enters the myocyte through slow channels, stimulation of the sarcoplasmic reticulum is diminished, myocardial contractions are weakened, and cardiac output declines. Drugs that improve myocardial contractility increase the amount of ionic calcium in the cytosol of myocytes. Digitalis and related compounds inhibit the sodium-potassium ATPase membrane pump and promote calcium influx through sodium exchange. β-Agonists stimulate the cardiac $\beta_1$-adrenergic receptors that provoke cAMP synthesis. Phosphodi-

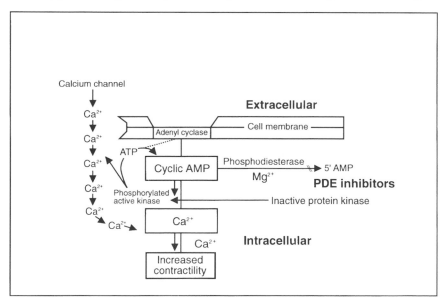

**FIGURE 9.**

Phosphodiesterase *(PDE)* III inhibitors increase myocardial contractility by limiting the degradation of cyclic adenosine monophosphate *(cAMP)*. *ATP* = adenosine triphosphate.

esterase inhibitors preserve cAMP by blocking the PDE III isoenzyme that is responsible for its degradation.[49]

The PDE inhibitors not only foster inotropy but also enhance lusitropy, i.e., ventricular relaxation that requires active calcium transport. For contractile proteins to relax, calcium must be actively pumped out of the cytosol, which also restores transmembrane potentials in preparation for the next depolarization event. Increases in cAMP levels in response to amrinone and milrinone accelerate calcium ion reuptake from the cytosol and also expulsion from the myocyte, thus assisting relaxation to improve filing.

In addition to their effect on the myocardium,[63] PDE inhibitors act peripherally as vasodilators and increase cAMP in vascular smooth muscle by inhibiting its metabolism.[64] When intracellular cAMP levels are increased, calcium uptake by the sarcoplasmic reticulum is augmented and less calcium is left for contraction. Smooth muscle relaxation and vasodilation result.[58]

The three major pharmacologic effects attributed to amrinone and milrinone—inotropy, lusitropy, and vasodilation—collectively produce an increase in cardiac output and reductions in right and left filling pressures and systemic vascular resistance.[65, 66] A left shift in the pressure-volume loop representing left ventricular systolic failure is accompanied by a downward shift that indicates reduced diastolic pressure at any given diastolic volume (Fig 10).

Milrinone has also been shown to decrease right-ventricular end-systolic volume and afterload as measured by pulmonary artery end-systolic pressure.[67] In patients with severe heart failure, milrinone improved the ejection fraction by approximately 25% by producing a decrease in end-systolic volume. The improvement in right ventricular performance was associated with a reduction in right ventricular afterload that was secondary to pulmonary vasodilation following milrinone infusion. The hemodynamic effects of the PDE inhibitors, i.e., improvement in cardiac output and a reduction in systemic vascular resistance and pulmonary capillary wedge pressure, occur without a concomitant increase in heart rate or myocardial oxygen demand.[68-70]

As with other cardiotonics, amrinone and milrinone have been compared with one another and with drugs from other therapeutic groups.[71-75] When hemodynamic responses to milrinone, nitroprusside, and dobutamine were assessed in patients with heart failure (Fig 11), differences in the actions of these drugs were noted.[49] Milrinone produced an increase in cardiac contractility following administration, whereas nitroprusside did not, as noted by changes in the rate of pressure rise during systole ($+dP/dt$) measured against

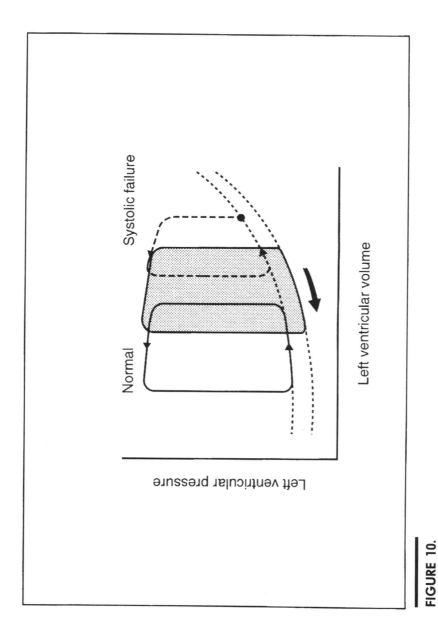

**FIGURE 10.**

The effects of milrinone on left ventricular pressure and volume during systolic pressure.

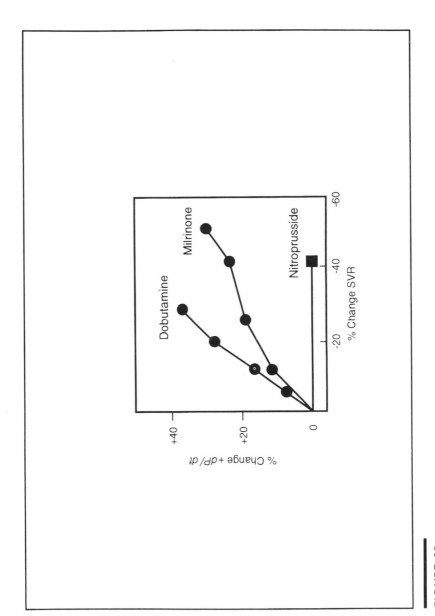

**FIGURE 11.**

Whereas dobutamine is predominantly inotropic and nitroprusside is solely vasodilatory, milrinone has effects on both cardiac contractility and vasculature dilation. (From Colucci WS, et al: *Circulation* 73(suppl 3):175–183, 1986. Used by permission.)

changes in systemic vascular resistance. By using the same parameters, milrinone produced a considerably greater reduction in arterial resistance as compared with dobutamine for all comparable levels of change in the rate of rise of systolic pressure (contractility). Dobutamine improved contractility to a slightly greater extent than milrinone did. These comparisons indicate that milrinone possesses a balance of inotropic and vasodilator properties that contribute to its clinical effects and distinguish it from pure vasodilators and pure inotropes.

Other comparisons indicate that amrinone and epinephrine produce similar increases in right ventricular stroke volume (16 and 13 mL per beat, respectively) when administered individually to patients following cardiopulmonary bypass.[76] When administered in combination, amrinone plus epinephrine increased stroke volume by 38 mL per beat, more than the sum total of their individual effects. This observation suggests that PDE inhibitors and β-agonists may have additive or synergistic effects when used in combination in postbypass patients. Supportive evidence for a combination effect resides in another study in which the combination of amrinone and dobutamine increased myocardial contractility ($+dP/dt$) and the cardiac index in patients with severe heart failure more than either drug alone.[77]

The benefits of any drug used in the treatment of acute heart failure must be weighed against the adverse effects associated with its use. The major concerns related to the surgical use of PDE inhibitors are hypotension, arrhythmias, and bleeding. As with any vasodilator, hypotension may follow the administration of either amrinone or milrinone, especially in patients who are hypovolemic. Hypotension has been associated more with amrinone than milrinone, but this observation may relate to the order of clinical availability, i.e., amrinone preceded milrinone by several years, and the relative inexperience of clinicians with a new class of drugs. The potential for hypotension, cited in clinical studies at less than 3% for milrinone, can be reduced by ensuring adequate patient hydration and administering a loading dose slowly over a couple of minutes.

In patients who are predisposed to arrhythmias, the administration of a drug with inotropic properties can precipitate an adverse event. Although the likelihood of serious arrhythmias is low (8.5% ventricular ectopic activity, 2.8% nonsustained ventricular tachycardia, 1.0% sustained ventricular tachycardia, and 0.1% ventricular fibrillation for milrinone) and intervention is not usually required, caution is advised whenever cardiotonic drugs are given.

In a milrinone-dobutamine comparative trial, the overall incidence of arrhythmias was 9.8% with milrinone and 15.4% with dobutamine. Nonsustained ventricular tachycardia occurred in two patients from each group, whereas sustained ventricular tachycardia occurred in one patient and ventricular fibrillation occurred in another patient in the milrinone-treated group.

The effect of PDE inhibitors on platelets tends to slow their aggregation in response to various stimuli. Additionally, thrombocytopenia (platelet count below 100,000/mm$^3$ or normal limits) has been recorded in 2.4% of patients receiving amrinone and appears to be related to a decrease in survival time as a consequence of splenic trapping. Thrombocytopenia has not been observed with milrinone, and bleeding phenomena have not been noted.

## CONSIDERATIONS THAT HAVE AN IMPACT ON THERAPEUTIC SELECTIONS

When the physiologic actions of inotropic agents were reviewed, obscured in data available from the literature was the significant variability that may exist from one patient to another. Moreover, in patients the actions of a drug are the combination of the intrinsic drug action and the secondary physiologic (automonic) response that accompanies it. For example, norepinephrine tends to increase the contractile rate of isolated myocytes in vitro, but in vivo, the potent $\alpha_1$-agonist effect and $\beta_1$-contractile effect raise blood pressure in healthy individuals and produce reflux bradycardia. In the same fashion, drugs given to patients with limitations in their ability to respond to certain actions may produce undesirable effects. Epinephrine has both $\alpha_1$ and $\beta_1$ action. In patients experiencing downregulation of $\beta_1$ receptors or in those who are receiving selective β-blocking drugs, the predominant effect seen may be increased systemic vascular resistance and decreased cardiac output. The same may be true in patients with significant myofibrosis and a severe reduction in ejection fraction. Awareness of such interrelationships is critical when choosing therapies to augment cardiac output.

### DOWNREGULATION OF β RECEPTORS

During heart failure a series of compensatory mechanisms adjust hemodynamics to maintain cardiac output and systemic perfusion. Enhanced catecholamine release from the adrenal medulla and sympathetic nerves leads to increased β receptor stimulation in the heart, a positive inotropic effect, and tachycardia. Peripheral vasoconstriction completes the picture of sympathetic stimulation.

With β stimulation of the heart, however, comes a reduction in the sensitivity (downregulation) and density of β-adrenergic receptors.[78] This functional and structural diminishment blunts the heart's response to catecholamines, which leads to further decreases in contractility and cardiac output (Fig 12). It also limits the therapeutic efficacy of sympathomimetic agents, but not PDE inhibitors, that are used before, during, and after surgery. Phosphodiesterase inhibitors circumvent β downregulation because of their receptor-independent actions.

## MYOCARDIAL ISCHEMIA AND INFARCTION

Patients with a history of recent or past myocardial infarction and limited coronary perfusion present a formidable challenge during cardiac surgery. Prone to acute failure and additional ischemic injury, these patients often require pharmacologic assistance to enhance their cardiac performance but are vulnerable to increases in heart rate and wall stress that heighten myocardial oxygen demand. In this circumstance, the selected agent or agents should improve cardiac output without increasing oxygen consumption. Improving contractile force is desirable, and unloading the heart is beneficial. The combined use of an inotrope and a vasodilator may improve

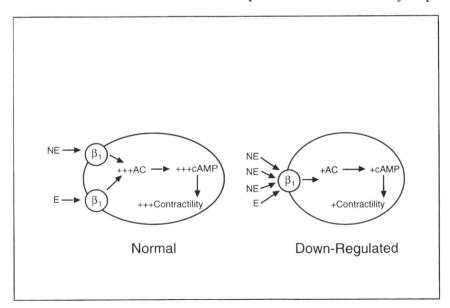

**FIGURE 12.**
Activation of β receptors results in downregulation and a blunted response to drug stimulation. *NE* = norepinephrine; *E* = epinephrine.

stroke volume by increasing contractility and reducing impedance with little change in myocardial oxygen consumption. The same objectives can be achieved with an inodilator such as amrinone or milrinone, both of which have been shown to have minimal effects on mean ventricular oxygen consumption yet substantially increase cardiac output in this setting.[68, 71, 75]

## SYSTOLIC VS. DIASTOLIC DYSFUNCTION

Ventricular ischemia impairs not only contractility but also distensibility[79] and is a primary cause of heart failure. Methods to improve the performance of a failing heart, however, usually focus on amelioration of systolic dysfunction and frequently overlook diastolic dysfunction, which may be a critical contributing factor to the failure and the predominant factor in patients with restrictive failure.[80-83] Combined dysfunction results in a decrease in stroke volume and an increase in left ventricular end-diastolic pressure, two problems that require correction if cardiac performance is to be improved. Consequently, therapeutic intervention should address these abnormalities as well as the impairment in contractility. Drugs that increase cAMP in the heart, the sympathomimetics and PDE inhibitors, have inotropic and lusitropic effects as long as their modes of action are not thwarted by hypocalcemia or β-blockage, which could be pharmacologic, functional, or structural.

## RESPONSIVENESS OF STUNNED MYOCARDIUM

Myocardial stunning is a reversible phenomenon that arises after reperfusion of ischemic myocardium. Its proposed cause is a decrease in the sensitivity of the myocytic contractile apparatus to ionic calcium secondary to the loss of energy-rich phosphates during ischemia.[84] Although not associated with myocardial necrosis, the contractile abnormalities that are characteristic of stunning can persist for days and compromise ventricular performance.[85-87] One important property of stunned myocardium is retention of the response to inotropic stimulation. Dopamine,[88] epinephrine,[89] isoproterenol,[90] dobutamine,[88] amrinone, and milrinone have the ability to elicit inotropic responses from stunned myocardium. However, it is not known whether full contractile reserve exists in the stunned tissue.

## CONSEQUENCES OF FAILING TO SEPARATE FROM CARDIOPULMONARY BYPASS

Failure to separate from cardiopulmonary bypass initiates a downward spiral in hemodynamics that contributes to the morbidity and mortality of cardiac surgery. If the initial attempt to separate fails, already diminished ventricular function worsens, contractions become less forceful, distension mounts, and wall stress increases. These unfavorable conditions increase oxygen demand yet reduce cardiac perfusion, thus creating additional ischemia and further reductions in contractility and overall performance. This imbalance in myocardial demand and delivery may produce secondary stunning and render subsequent attempts to terminate bypass more difficult. Difficulty separating from bypass also increases pump time and the probability that red blood cells, platelets, and coagulation factors will be damaged. If failure is imminent during any attempt to separate, reinstitution of bypass can prevent the added functional deterioration and systemic hypotension that can jeopardize vital perfusion. If failure occurs postoperatively after initially successful weaning, reheparinization and return to bypass may be required.[15] In addition to the detrimental effects on the heart, failed weaning may lead to neurologic sequelae, organ damage, adverse hematologic events, and occasionally death. The cost associated with added bypass time or the use of mechanical assist devices, although secondary to the well-being of the patient, is yet another concern. All of these factors are central to the timing of pharmacologic intervention for cardiac patients in critical settings and lead some physicians to use cardiotonic drugs prophylactically in an attempt to separate patients from cardiopulmonary bypass. Early intervention may circumvent the downhill spiral of failed weaning.

Drugs that potentiate the heart's performance with increased contractility augment output at a critical point in the course of surgery and facilitate separation from bypass. Diastolic function should also be enhanced because decreased relaxation and compliance follow reperfusion and can lower cardiac output.[91] Right heart performance should be supported as well. The overall objective is to ensure, as much as possible, successful separation from bypass on the first attempt, avoid the need for intra-aortic balloon pumping (particularly for patients with severe peripheral vascular disease), and prevent a postoperative deterioration that necessitates reinstitution of bypass.[15]

## CAVEATS IN THE MANAGEMENT OF ACUTE LOW CARDIAC OUTPUT STATES

The management of patients with acute heart failure and acute low cardiac output states requires a balance of clinical acumen and scientific knowledge. Clinicians must also anticipate potential future problems that their patients may experience and attempt to prevent them. Treatment of the patient, not just the heart, is paramount to successful clinical outcomes. It is interesting to consider cardiac surgical patients requiring inotropic support in perspective. According to the New York Heart Association classification, most patients requiring perioperative support are physiologically similar to those with class III or, more often, class IV failure. These patients are very sensitive to the adverse effects of increased systemic vascular resistance on cardiac performance, but at times the cardiac index may have to be rendered secondary to perfusion pressures compatible with adequate cerebral and coronary perfusion.

## REFERENCES

1. Royster RL: Myocardial dysfunction following cardiopulmonary bypass: Recovery patterns, predictors of inotropic need, theoretical concepts of inotropic administration. *J Cardiothorac Vasc Anesth* 7(suppl 2):19–25, 1993.
2. Cohn PF, Gorlin R, Cohn LH, et al: Left ventricular ejection fraction as a prognostic guide in surgical treatment of coronary and valvular heart disease. *Am J Cardiol* 34:136–141, 1974.
3. Nelson GR, Cohn PF, Gorlin R: Prognosis in medically treated coronary artery disease: Influence of ejection fraction compared to other parameters. *Circulation* 52:408–412, 1975.
4. Gersh BJ, Kronmal RA, Frye RL, et al: Coronary anteriography and coronary artery bypass surgery: Morbidity and mortality in patients 65 years or older. A report from the Coronary Artery Surgery Study. *Circulation* 67:483–491, 1983.
5. Royster RL, Butterworth JF IV, Prough DS, et al: Preoperative and intraoperative predictors of inotropic support and long-term outcome in patients having coronary artery bypass grafting. *Anesth Analg* 72:153–185, 1991.
6. Mangano DT: Perioperative cardiac morbidity. *Anesthesiology* 72:153–185, 1990.
7. Breisblatt WM, Stein KL, Wolfe CJ, et al: Acute myocardial dysfunction and recovery: A common occurrence after coronary bypass surgery. *J Am Coll Cardiol* 15:1261–1269, 1990.
8. Gray R, Maddahi J, Berman D, et al: Scintigraphic and hemodynamic demonstration of transient left ventricular dysfunction immediately after uncomplicated coronary artery bypass grafting. *J Thorac Cardiovasc Surg* 77:504–510, 1979.
9. Roberts M, Spies SM, Meyers SN, et al: Early and long-term improvement in left ventricular performance following coronary bypass surgery. *Surgery* 88:467–475, 1980.
10. Phillips HR, Carter JE, Okada RD, et al: Serial changes in left ventricu-

lar ejection fraction in the early hours after aortocoronary bypass grafting. *Chest* 83:28–34, 1983.

11. Sell TL, Purut CM, Silva R, et al: Recovery of myocardial function during coronary artery bypass grafting: Intraoperative assessment by pressure-volume loops. *J Thorac Cardiovasc Surg* 101:681–687, 1991.

12. Mintz LJ, Ingels NB Jr, Daughters GT II, et al: Sequential studies of left ventricular function and wall motion after coronary arterial bypass surgery. *Am J Cardiol* 45:210–216, 1980.

13. Schlant RC, Sonnenblick EH: Pathophysiology of heart failure, in Schlant RC, Alexander RW (eds): *Hurst's The Heart: Arteries and Veins.* New York, McGraw-Hill, 1994.

14. Cheitlin MD, Sokolow M, McIlroy MB: *Clinical Cardiology.* E Norwalk, Conn, Appleton & Lange, 1993.

15. Lewis KP: Early intervention of inotropic support in facilitating weaning from cardiopulmonary bypass: The New England Deaconess Hospital experience. *J Cardiothorac Vasc Anesth* 7(suppl 2):40–45, 1993.

16. d'Hollander A, Primo G, Hennart D, et al: Compared efficacy of dobutamine and dopamine in association with calcium chloride on termination of cardiopulmonary bypass. *J Thorac Cardiovasc Surg* 83:264–271, 1982.

17. Hosking MP: Should calcium be administered prior to separation from cardiopulmonary bypass? *Anesthesiology* 75:1121–1122, 1991.

18. Koski G: Con: Calcium salts are contraindicated in weaning of patients from cardiopulmonary bypass after coronary artery surgery. *J Cardiothorac Anesth* 2:570–575, 1988.

19. Fernandez-del Castillo C, Harringer W, Warshaw AL, et al: Risk factors for pancreatic cellular injury after cardiopulmonary bypass. *N Engl J Med* 325:382–387, 1991.

20. Butterworth JF IV, Royster RL, Prielipp RC, et al: In reply: Hosking MP. Should calcium be administered prior to separation from cardiopulmonary bypass? *Anesthesiology* 75:1121–1122, 1991.

21. Butterworth JF IV, Strickland RA, Mark LJ, et al: Calcium does not augment phenylephrine's hypertensive effects. *Crit Care Med* 18:603–606, 1990.

22. Butterworth JF IV, Strickland RA, Zaloga GP: Hemodynamic actions and drug interactions of calcium and magnesium, in Zaloga GP (ed): *Problems in Critical Care,* vol 4. Philadelphia, JB Lippincott, 1990, pp 402–415.

23. Zaloga GP, Strickland RA, Butterworth JF IV, et al: Calcium attenuates epinephrine's beta-adrenergic effects in postoperative heart surgery patients. *Circulation* 81:196–200, 1990.

24. Royster RL, Butterworth JF IV, Prielipp RC, et al: A randomized, blinded, placebo-controlled evaluation of calcium chloride and epinephrine for inotropic support after emergence from cardiopulmonary bypass. *Anesth Analg* 74:3–13, 1992.

25. Robertie PG, Butterworth JF IV, Royster RL, et al: Normal parathyroid

hormone responses to hypocalcemia during cardiopulmonary bypass. *Anesthesiology* 75:43–48, 1991.

26. Marban E, Koretsune Y, Corretti M, et al: Calcium and its role in myo-cardial cell injury during ischemia and reperfusion. *Circulation* 80(suppl 4):17–22, 1989.

27. Butterworth JF IV, Zaloga GP, Prielipp RC, et al: Calcium inhibits the cardiac stimulating properties of dobutamine but not of amrinone. *Chest* 101:174–180, 1992.

28. Gerber JG, Nies AS: Antihypertensive agents and the drug therapy of hypertension, in Gilman AG, Rall TW, Nies AW, et al (eds): *The Pharmacological Basis of Therapeutics*, ed 8. New York, Pergamon Press, 1990, pp 784–813.

29. Rapoport RM, Murad F: Endothelium-dependent and nitrovasodilator-induced relaxation of vascular smooth muscle: Role for cyclic GMP. *J Cyclic Nucleotide Protein Phosphor Res* 9:281–296, 1983.

30. Murad F: Cyclic guanosine monophosphate as a mediator of vasodilation. *J Clin Invest* 78:1–5, 1986.

31. Cohn JN, Burke LP: Nitroprusside. *Ann Intern Med* 91:752–757, 1979.

32. Waldman SA, Murad F: Cyclic GMP synthesis and function. *Pharmacol Rev* 39:163–196, 1987.

33. *Physicians' Desk Reference*. Orddell, NJ, Medical Economics, 1995.

34. Moncada S, Radomski MW, Palmer RM: Endothelium-derived relaxing factor. Identification as nitric oxide and role in the control of vascular tone and platelet function. *Biochem Pharmacol* 37:2495–2501, 1988.

35. McEvoy GK (ed): *AHFS Drug Information*. Bethesda, Md, American Society of Health-System Pharmacists, 1995.

36. Wilkins RW, Haynes FW, Weiss S: The role of the venous system in the circulatory collapse induced by sodium nitrite. *J Clin Invest* 85:85–91, 1937.

37. Mason DJ, Braunwald EB: The effects of nitroglycerin and amylnitrite on arteriolar and venous tone in the human forearm. *Circulation* 32:755–766, 1965.

38. Kamijo T, Tomaru T, Miwa AY, et al: The effects of dobutamine, propranolol, and nitroglycerin on an experimental canine model of congestive heart failure. *Jpn J Pharmacol* 65:223–231, 1994.

39. Ghio S, Poli A, Farrario M, et al: Haemodynamic effects of glyceryl trinitrate during continuous 24 hour infusion in patients with heart failure. *Br Heart J* 72:145–149, 1994.

40. Ivankovich AD, Miletich DJ, Albrecht RF, et al: Sodium nitroprusside and cerebral blood flow in the anesthetized and unanesthetized goat. *Anesthesiology* 44:21–26, 1976.

41. Pace JB: Pulmonary vascular response to sodium nitroprusside in anesthetized dogs. *Anesth Analg* 57:551–557, 1978.

42. Chiariello M, Gold HK, Leinbach RC, et al: Comparison between the

effects of nitroprusside and nitroglycerin on ischemic injury during acute myocardial infarction. *Circulation* 54:766–773, 1976.

43. Awan NA, Miller RR, Vera Z, et al: Reduction of ST segment elevation with infusion of nitroprusside in patients with acute myocardial infarction. *Am J Cardiol* 38:435–439, 1976.

44. Cohn JN, Franciosa JA, Francis GS, et al: Effect of short-term infusion of sodium nitroprusside on mortality rate in acute myocardial infarction complicated by left ventricular failure: Results of a Veterans Administration cooperative study. *N Engl J Med* 306:1129–1135, 1982.

45. McDowall DG, Keaney NP, Turner JM, et al: The toxicity of sodium nitroprusside. *Br J Anaesth* 46:327–332, 1974.

46. Ahlquist RP: A study of the adrenotropic receptors. *Am J Physiol* 153:586–600, 1948.

47. Hoffman BB, Lefkowitz RJ: Alpha-adrenergic receptor subtypes. *N Engl J Med* 302:1390–1396, 1980.

48. Scheuer J, Bhan AK: Cardiac contractile proteins. Adenosine triphosphatase activity and physiological function. *Circ Res* 45:1–12, 1979.

49. Colucci WS, Wright RF, Braunwald E: New positive inotropic agents in the treatment of congestive heart failure. *N Engl J Med* 314:290–299, 1986.

50. LeJemtel TH, Sonnenblick EH: Nonglycosidic cardioactive agents, in Schlant RC, Alexander RW (eds): *Hurst's The Heart: Arteries and Veins.* New York, McGraw-Hill, 1994.

51. DiSesa VJ, Brown E, Mudge GH Jr, et al: Hemodynamic comparison of dopamine and dobutamine in the postoperative volume-loaded, pressure-loaded and normal ventricle. *J Thorac Cardiovasc Surg* 83:256–263, 1982.

52. Fowler MB, Alderman EL, Oesterle SN, et al: Dobutamine and dopamine after cardiac surgery: Greater augmentation of myocardial blood flow with dobutamine. *Circulation* 70(suppl 1):103–111, 1984.

53. Salomon NW, Plachetka JR, Copeland JG: Comparison of dopamine and dobutamine following coronary artery bypass grafting. *Ann Thorac Surg* 33:48–54, 1982.

54. Steen PA, Tinker JH, Pluth JR, et al: Efficacy of dopamine, dobutamine, and epinephrine during emergence from cardiopulmonary bypass in man. *Circulation* 57:378–384, 1978.

55. Royster RL: Intraoperative administration of inotropes in cardiac surgery patients. *J Cardiothorac Anesth* 4:17–28, 1990.

56. Butterworth JF IV, Prielipp RC, Zaloga GP, et al: Is dobutamine less chronotropic than epinephrine after coronary bypass surgery (abstract)? *Anesthesiology* 73:61, 1990.

57. Sonnenblick EH, Frishman WH, LeJemtel TH: Dobutamine: A new synthetic cardioactive sympathetic amine. *N Engl J Med* 300:17–22, 1979.

58. Smith TW, Braunwald E, Kelly RA: The management of heart failure,

in Braunwald E (ed): *Heart Disease. A Textbook of Cardiovascular Medicine.* Philadelphia, WB Saunders; 1992, pp 464–519.

59. Williams RS, Bishop T: Selectivity of dobutamine for adrenergic receptor subtypes: In vitro analysis by radioligand binding. *J Clin Invest* 67:1703–1711, 1981.
60. Tyden H, Nystrom SO: Dopamine versus dobutamine after open-heart surgery. *Acta Anaesthesiol Scand* 27:193–198, 1983.
61. Sethna DH, Gray RJ, Moffitt EA, et al: Dobutamine and cardiac oxygen balance in patients following myocardial revascularization. *Anesth Analg* 61:917–920, 1982.
62. Vatner SF, Baig H: Importance of heart rate in determining the effects of sympathomimetic amines on regional myocardial function and blood flow in conscious dogs with acute myocardial ischemia. *Circ Res* 45:793–803, 1979.
63. Sonnenblick EH, Grose R, Strain J, et al: Effects of milrinone on left ventricular performance and myocardial contractility in patients with severe heart failure. *Circulation* 73(suppl 3):162–167, 1986.
64. Evans DB: Overview of cardiovascular physiologic and pharmacologic aspects of selective phosphodiesterase peak III inhibitors. *Am J Cardiol* 63:9A–11A, 1989.
65. Anderson JL: Hemodynamic and clinical benefits with intravenous milrinone in severe chronic heart failure: Results of a multicenter study in the United States. *Am Heart J* 121:1956–1964, 1991.
66. Baim DS, McDowell AV, Cherniles J, et al: Evaluation of a new bipyridine inotropic agent—milrinone—in patients with severe congestive heart failure. *N Engl J Med* 309:748–756, 1983.
67. Eichhorn EJ, Konstam MA, Weiland DS, et al: Differential effects of milrinone and dobutamine on right ventricular preload, afterload and systolic performance in congestive heart failure secondary to ischemic or idiopathic dilated cardiomyopathy. *Am J Cardiol* 60:1329–1333, 1987.
68. Monrad ES, Baim DS, Smith HS, et al: Effects of milrinone on coronary hemodynamics and myocardial energetics in patients with congestive heart failure. *Circulation* 71:972–979, 1985.
69. Benotti JR, Grossman W, Braunwald E, et al: Effects of amrinone on myocardial energy metabolism and hemodynamics in patients with severe congestive heart failure due to coronary artery disease. *Circulation* 62:28–34, 1980.
70. Chatterjee K: Digitalis, catecholamines, and other positive inotropic agents, in Chatterjee K, Parmley WW (eds): *Cardiology, Physiology, Pharmacology, Diagnosis.* Philadelphia, JB Lippincott, 1991, pp 234–274.
71. Monrad ES, Baim DS, Smith HS, et al: Milrinone, dobutamine, and nitroprusside: Comparative effects on hemodynamics and myocardial energetics in patients with severe congestive heart failure. *Circulation* 73(suppl 3):168–174, 1986.

72. Biddle TL, Benotti JR, Creager MA, et al: Comparison of intravenous milrinone and dobutamine for congestive heart failure secondary to either ischemic or dilated cardiomyopathy. *Am J Cardiol* 59:1345–1350, 1987.

73. Jaski BE, Fifer MA, Wright RF, et al: Positive inotropic and vasodilator actions of milrinone in patients with severe congestive heart failure: Dose-response relationships and comparison to nitroprusside. *J Clin Invest* 75:643–649, 1985.

74. Colucci WS, Denniss AR, Leatherman GF, et al: Intracoronary infusion of dobutamine to patients with and without severe congestive heart failure: Dose-response relationships, correlation with circulating catecholamines, and the effect of phosphodiesterase inhibition. *J Clin Invest* 81:1103–1110, 1988.

75. Grose R, Strain J, Greenberg M, et al: Systemic and coronary effects of intravenous milrinone and dobutamine in congestive heart failure. *J Am Coll Cardiol* 7:1107–1113, 1986.

76. Royster RL, Butterworth JF IV, Prielipp RC, et al: A randomized, blinded trial of amrinone, epinephrine, and amrinone/epinephrine after cardiopulmonary bypass (CPB) (abstract). *Anesthesiology* 75:148, 1991.

77. Gage J, Rutman H, Lucido D, et al: Additive effects of dobutamine and amrinone on myocardial contractility and ventricular performance in patients with severe heart failure. *Circulation* 74:367–373, 1986.

78. Bristow MR, Port JD, Hershberger RE, et al: The β-adrenergic receptor–adenylate cyclase complex as a target for therapeutic intervention in heart failure. *Eur Heart J* 10(suppl B):45–54, 1989.

79. Perret C: Acute heart failure in myocardial infarction: Principles of treatment. *Crit Care Med* 18(suppl):26–29, 1990.

80. Lew WY: Evaluation of left ventricular diastolic function. *Circulation* 79:1393–1397, 1989.

81. Packer M: Diastolic function as a target of therapeutic interventions in chronic heart failure. *Eur Heart J* 11(suppl C):35–40, 1990.

82. Stauffer JC, Gaasch WH: Recognition and treatment of left ventricular diastolic dysfunction. *Prog Cardiovasc Dis* 32:319–332, 1990.

83. Dougherty AH, Naccarelli GV, Gray EL, et al: Congestive heart failure with normal systolic function. *Am J Cardiol* 54:778–782, 1984.

84. Swain JL, Sabina RL, McHale PA, et al: Prolonged myocardial nucleotide depletion after brief ischemia in the open-chest dog. *Am J Physiol* 242:H818–H826, 1982.

85. Heyndrickx GR, Millard RW, McRitchie RJ, et al: Regional myocardial functional and electrophysiological alterations after brief coronary artery occlusion in conscious dogs. *J Clin Invest* 56:978–985, 1975.

86. Theroux P, Ross J Jr, Franklin D, et al: Coronary arterial reperfusion. III. Early and late effects on regional myocardial function and dimensions in conscious dogs. *Am J Cardiol* 38:599–606, 1976.

87. Weiner JM, Astein CS, Arthur JH, et al: Persistence of myocardial in-

jury following brief periods of coronary occlusion. *Cardiovasc Res* 10:678–686, 1976.

88. Ellis SG, Wynne J, Braunwald E, et al: Response of reperfusion-salvaged, stunned myocardium to inotropic stimulation. *Am Heart J* 107:13–19, 1984.
89. Becker LC, Levine JH, DiPaula AF, et al: Reversal of dysfunction in postischemic stunned myocardium by epinephrine and postextrasystolic potentiation. *J AM Coll Cardiol* 7:580–589, 1986.
90. Bolli R, Zhu WX, Myers ML, et al: Beta-adrenergic stimulation reverses postischemic myocardial dysfunction without producing subsequent functional deterioration. *Am J Cardiol* 56:964–968, 1985.
91. Ehring T, Schulz R, Schipke JD, et al: Diastolic dysfunction of stunned myocardium. *Am J Cardiol Pathol* 4:358–366, 1993.

# Aortic Valve Reparative Procedures

### Charles D. Fraser, Jr., M.D.

Cleveland Clinic Foundation, Department of Thoracic and
Cardiovascular Surgery, Cleveland, Ohio

### Delos M. Cosgrove III, M.D.

Cleveland Clinic Foundation, Department of Thoracic and
Cardiovascular Surgery, Cleveland, Ohio

A ortic valve repair was one of the first open intracardiac procedures attempted. Although the initial results were somewhat encouraging, this approach to the treatment of aortic valve disease was largely abandoned after the introduction of safe valve prostheses.[1–5] Indeed, the development and widespread clinical application of both mechanical and bioprosthetic valves rank as one of the real success stories of modern cardiac surgery. The era of reliable mechanical valve prostheses was initiated after the development of the Starr-Edwards ball-and-cage valve in the early 1960s.[6] Concurrent developments in New Zealand and England by Barratt-Boyes and Ross, respectively, demonstrated the utility of homograft or allograft valves for aortic valve replacement.[7, 8] Tremendous advances in structural integrity and biocompatibility occurred over the ensuing decades so that in the current era the cardiac surgeon has a variety of mechanical and bioprosthetic valve options available in the treatment of an individual patient. More recently, a resurgence in interest in the use of autologous, pulmonary homograft tissue transplants to the aortic position by using the so-called Ross procedure, after its developer, Sir Donald Ross, added yet another option to the surgical armamentarium.[9, 10]

Considerable data are available to support the relative safety of aortic valve replacement in a variety of clinical settings.[11, 12] Furthermore, detailed follow-up data exist for all varieties of prosthetic and biological valves currently in use, so surgeons and cardiologists can have a reasonable degree of accuracy in predicting the long-term risks associated with each option in an individual patient. Overall, the long-term risks associated with having some form of aortic valve replacement have been documented to be relatively low. The degree of ongoing risk in an individual patient clearly relates to a constellation of factors, including the type of prosthesis, the necessity for anticoagulation, age, and associated co-morbid factors such as coronary artery disease and ventricular function.[13-24] Complications associated with lifelong valvular prostheses may include mechanical failure, thromboembolism, endocarditis, hemolysis, paravalvular leakage, and anticoagulant-related hemorrhage. Although the likelihood of any one prosthesis-related complication is low, an individual may still be at some significant lifetime risk when faced with many years of living with a prosthetic aortic valve.

After consideration of the ongoing risk associated with aortic valve replacement, we have re-examined the possibility of repairing aortic valves in selected patients with appropriate pathology. Our hypothesis has been that in patients with certain types of aortic valve pathology, successful valve repair may afford the individual the opportunity of lower risks of complications associated with having one's own native aortic valve. We have felt particularly compelled to use these techniques in young individuals facing the necessity of aortic valve surgery. In such patients, the potential long duration of needing a valve prosthesis combined with issues regarding lifestyle, desire for childbearing, and level of maturity have led us to work very hard to preserve the patient's native aortic valve if possible. Further, our increasing level of comfort with cardiac reoperations combined with the relative safety of such procedures has encouraged us to choose valve repair as a palliative intermediate-term step rather than a bioprosthesis in certain young patients.[24]

At present, we consider aortic valve repair to be a viable option for certain types of pathology to be described later. Although the long-term results are as yet unknown, our short- and intermediate-term data are encouraging.

## AORTIC VALVE PATHOLOGY

### INSUFFICIENT BICUSPID AORTIC VALVES

A bicuspid aortic valve is the most commonly recognized congenital cardiac morphologic anomaly. Although not precisely known, the prevalence of this anomaly has been estimated to be up to 2% in the general population.[25, 26] The majority of patients born with a bicuspid aortic valve live a normal life span without a pathologic process developing in association with their congenital cardiac anomaly.[27] In repairing bicuspid aortic valves, it has been our desire to return our patients to this population of individuals.

The pathologic processes associated with a congenitally bicuspid aortic valve may result in aortic insufficiency, stenosis, or both. The vast majority of our patients undergoing reparative aortic valve surgery have had insufficient bicuspid aortic valves secondary to cusp prolapse. As has been eloquently described by Willcox and Anderson, in a normal heart the aortic cusps have deep "semilunar" attachments at their hinge points.[28] This area is commonly referred to as the aortic annulus, but indeed it is not truly an annulus because it is not circular in appearance, nor do the points of attachment all lie in the same vertical plane. The intercusp triangles are long and narrow in normal valves. This provides a broad zone of leaflet coaptation or lunula. In a normally functioning aortic valve, whether bicuspid or tricuspid, the central load-bearing area of the cusp is supported during valve closure by the lunula or area of coaptation and the valve commissures. The cusps meet at the lead point on the edge of the valve leaflet, which is identifiable as a slightly thickened area known as the nodule of Arantius.

The elegant mechanism of properly functioning aortic valves has long been a source of intrigue and study, indeed dating at least back to the days of Leonardo da Vinci. To date, the most complete investigation of the structural and mechanical function of the aortic valve is found in the outstanding monograph on the subject produced by Mano Thubrikar.[29] Dr. Thubrikar's work has provided considerable understanding not only in the proper functioning of normal aortic valves but also in designing reparative techniques to attempt to reconstruct physiologic valve function. As mentioned earlier, normal aortic valves have deep, semilunar cusps. Tall, narrow interleaflet triangles have their apices at the aortic valve commissures. The height and width of the interleaflet triangle governs the area of cusp apposition or lunula. The lunula plays a critical role in determining the amount of load an individual cusp can support. The load-bearing area of the cusp has its load point at the nodule of Arantius.[30, 31]

In congenitally bicuspid aortic valves, several mechanisms may exist that result in valve insufficiency. In most bicuspid aortic valves, morphologic evaluation will demonstrate what appears to be failure of separation of two cusps. This most commonly occurs between what would have been the right and left coronary cusps.[32] In such cases, there often appears to be a rudimentary commissure that bisects the conjoined leaflet. This primitive commissure or raphe may be the source of restricted leaflet motion and or calcification (Fig 1).

The conjoined leaflet may have either an anteroposterior or right-left orientation. In insufficient valves, there is usually con-

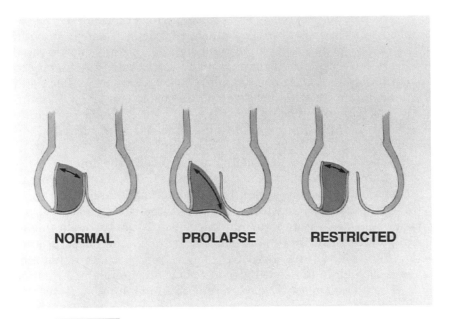

**NORMAL**          **PROLAPSE**          **RESTRICTED**

**FIGURE 1.**

Schematic representation of potential mechanisms for aortic valve insufficiency, including leaflet prolapse and restriction.

joined cusp prolapse. The free edge of the conjoined cusp is usually longer and thickened in comparison to the opposing cusp. There are often areas of fibrous thickening along the free edge of the prolapsing cusp. It has been our impression that this thickening corresponds to the region of turbulent regurgitant flow. As such, it has been a useful marker in directing the mode of repair (to be described later) (Fig 2, A and B).

In a bicuspid valve, the region of cusp attachment is crescentic in appearance as compared with the nearly semicircular or semilunar attachments in a normal aortic valve. The crescentic shape of the cusp attachment in a bicuspid valve results in a short, broad interleaflet triangle. Because the height of the interleaflet triangle is central to the area of leaflet coaptation, the relative degree of load-bearing capability of the cusp is decreased in a bicuspid valve. This fact, in combination with increased length of the conjoined cusp, predisposes some bicuspid aortic valves to insufficiency[32, 33] (Fig 3).

Patients with bicuspid aortic valves are also known to be at increased risk of bacterial endocarditis. Such an infection can lead to significant cusp perforations. In cases of resolved endocarditis, these perforations may be amenable to repair.

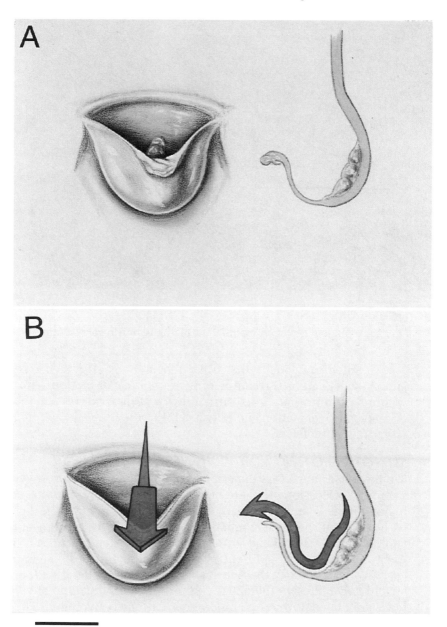

**FIGURE 2.**

In bicuspid valves, thickening of the raphe results in cusp restriction, and prolapse occurs secondary to excessive cusp length **(A)**. The mechanism of regurgitation results in a jet along the prolapsing segment with subsequent leaflet thickening in this area **(B)**.

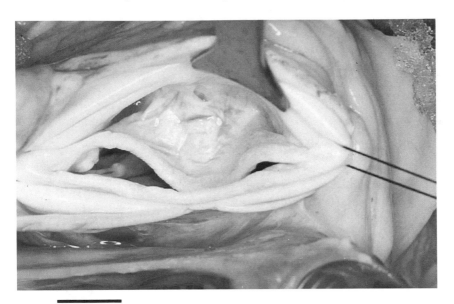

**FIGURE 3.**

Operative photograph of an insufficient bicuspid aortic valve. Note the excessive size of the conjoined cusp and obvious area of prolapse.

As noted previously, the raphe that may exist with the conjoined leaflet can be the source of restricted leaflet motion with or without calcification. This situation may also exacerbate inadequate leaflet coaptation and play a central role in the development of aortic insufficiency.

## STENOTIC BICUSPID AORTIC VALVES

We have had much less experience with this form of aortic valve pathology. Occasionally there may be some degree of commissural fusion that is potentially amenable to open valvotomy. This sort of pathology will be most frequently seen in the area of congenital cardiac defects associated with critical aortic stenosis presenting early in life. It may represent part of the spectrum of congenital aortic valve pathology that may range to a severely deformed, unicuspid valve. Present therapeutic approaches for this type of valve have gravitated toward percutaneous balloon valvotomy. Those critical cases requiring surgical therapy are often seen in newborns or small infants and as such as are most appropriately managed by a congenital cardiac surgeon. In general, little can be done to repair these valves, and successful surgical management may require aortic root replacement with either a homograft or autograph (Ross procedure). These techniques and the management of this category of patients are beyond the scope of this chapter and will not be dealt with further.

## NONRHEUMATIC AORTIC INSUFFICIENCY

Aortic root enlargement may be isolated or associated with a variety of connective tissue disorders, including Marfan syndrome resulting in annulo-aortic ectasia. In these conditions, the aortic valve is often morphologically normal. Central or eccentric aortic regurgitation develops with progressive root enlargement as the cusps are drawn apart and are no longer able to coapt properly.

In these conditions it is often quite tempting to attempt to preserve the native aortic valve. Although the cusps are usually normal, achieving valvar competence in this setting cannot be realized without a reduction in annular dimension. In patients with coexistent aneurysmal changes of the sinus portion of the ascending aorta, valve repair must be incorporated into some sort of root replacement. David and Feindel have championed such a technique that has come to be recognized as the "David" procedure.[34] Although we have used this technique with some success, it has not proved as reliable in our hands as the more proven and widely used composite root replacement as first described by Bentall and DeBono and widely applied by Gott and others to patients with annulo-aortic ectasia.[35, 36]

Patients with annular dilatation not associated with concomitant aneurysmal changes also represent a surgical challenge if repair is considered. With massive annular dilation without significant cusp prolapse, annular reduction is required if competence of the native valve is to be achieved. Techniques of annular plication have been used in cardiac surgery since the earliest days of attempted valve repair.[3–5, 37] More recently, Carpentier and colleagues have revisited these methods.[38] Annual plication using Carpentier's method requires a continuous, circular reduction of the annulus in an effort to promote improved cusp coaptation. We have had limited experience with this method and believe it to be too unpredictable in terms of reliability. Indeed, from Carpentier's reported series, the results are not particularly encouraging, with a 13% rate of need of early reoperation and 15% early incidence of moderate aortic insufficiency in the remaining patients.

A particularly interesting group of patients is represented by individuals with prolapse of a single cusp with or without an associated ventricular septal defect (VSD). This may occur with any aortic cusp but has been observed most frequently in either the right or noncoronary cusp. This observation has led some morphologists to hypothesize that some cases of leaflet prolapse may have had as their substrate a pre-existing subaortic VSD that spontaneously closed. Whatever the cause, these patients will often have otherwise normal aortic valves. Since many of these patients are quite young, we have felt compelled to attempt valve repair if possible in such cases.

An unrepaired subaortic VSD is frequently associated with aortic insufficiency secondary to cusp prolapse. Indeed, our policy regarding small VSDs that are otherwise not hemodynamically significant has been to close the VSD if we observe anything more than very mild aortic insufficiency. In patients with perimembranous-type VSDs, the prolapsing cusp is most commonly the noncoronary cusp. With outlet VSDs (also known as subarterial or supracristal VSDs), the right coronary cusp most frequently prolapses.[39, 40] In such cases, closing the VSD may or may not improve the aortic insufficiency. Decisions regarding concomitant valve repair relate to the severity of the insufficiency. As noted previously, this group of patients was one in which the earliest attempts at aortic valve repair were made as reported by Spencer, Trusler, and others.[3, 4]

## RHEUMATIC AORTIC INSUFFICIENCY

In patients suffering from rheumatic carditis and valvulitis, aortic insufficiency may occasionally develop very early in the course of their disease process. This is always associated with some sort of rheumatic mitral valve pathology. This sort of pathology will most frequently be seen in patients from areas with limited medical resources who have had inadequate treatment for their rheumatic disease. Often, such patients will be in a severely compromised state with severe aortic insufficiency and marked congestive heart failure. Patients in this situation should be considered beyond the confines of valve repair and should undergo valve replacement.

Other patients with rheumatic aortic insufficiency may have a much more insidious process with gradually progressive incompetence. In such individuals, the gross morphology of the valve may demonstrate thickening and infolding of the cusp edges resulting in central incompetence. The remainder of the valve may appear relatively normal with thin cusp bellies and unrestricted leaflet motion.[41, 42] These findings have led us and others to attempt valve repair in such patients. Our experience with repairing valves in this group has been limited and not wholly satisfactory. Duran has had considerable experience with this sort of patient and has described encouraging results with a technique of valve repair that employs leaflet extension using autologous pericardium (to be described later).[43]

## PATIENT EVALUATION/SELECTION
### PREOPERATIVE EVALUATION
As is clear from the preceding discussion, the majority of patients we select as potential candidates for aortic valve repair will suffer from aortic insufficiency secondary to cusp prolapse in either a bicuspid or tricuspid aortic valve. All of these patients will have had a preoperative echocardiogram (transthoracic and/or transesophageal) evaluation, including a color Doppler estimation of the severity of insufficiency. We have graded aortic insufficiency on a scale of 0 to 4 based on previously defined criteria as described by Perry and colleagues.[44] Valuable information concerning the aortic valve pathology can be gained at the hands of an experienced echocardiographer. Important morphologic data include the location of the aortic insufficiency (central vs. at the commissures), degree of leaflet prolapse, annular size, presence of a bicuspid or tricuspid arrangement, calcification, and presence of leaflet perforation. The echocardiographic study may also document coexisting structural or valvar pathology and may be used to estimate ventricular function.

We have not routinely required cardiac catheterization in patients without other suspected cardiac pathology. Clearly, patients with suspected coronary artery disease require cineangiography. Right and left heart catheterization with hemodynamic studies may prove useful in patients with other forms of associated cardiac pathology.

### PATIENT SELECTION
We have accepted patients for aortic valve repair who have moderate to severe aortic insufficiency associated with the appropriate pathology as described previously. The majority of our patients are young adults (the mean age in our series thus far is 39 years with a range of 15 to 68). We believe that these patients are most likely to realize the long-term advantages of having their native aortic valves preserved.

Controversy exists regarding the appropriate time to refer asymptomatic patients with aortic insufficiency for valve surgery. Clearly, in many instances this is of academic interest only because the decision to refer the patient for surgery may rest in the hands of the cardiologist, who may not have sought surgical input in the decision-making process. Admittedly, patients with moderate to sever aortic insufficiency may go for many years with relative preservation of left ventricular function. It appears that the prevailing attitude among cardiologists at this time is to follow such patients indefinitely while observing closely for evidence of a significant decline in ventricular function.[45] This tendency has been reinforced by recent reports indicating the efficacy of long-term vasodilator therapy with nifedipine in preserving ventricular function in asymptomatic patients with aortic insufficiency.[46]

Unfortunately, some young individuals may be "followed" for too long and suffer irreversible left ventricular dysfunction as the result of long-standing, severe aortic insufficiency. One such example is found in our series: a young man underwent successful valve repair only to go on to severe left ventricular dysfunction over the ensuing year, ultimately culminating in the necessity of cardiac transplantation. Several other patients with severely dilated ventricles at the time of successful repair continue to show ventricular dilation despite having competent valves.

These findings, combined with the safety of the procedure (no operative deaths in 108 consecutive patients), have led us to question whether patients with moderate to severe aortic insufficiency should be referred for surgery at an earlier time in the course of their disease. At present, patients with significant aortic insufficiency are examined very closely at the time they are first evaluated. This may include exercise testing and gated cardiac function studies in addition to precise echocardiographic determinations of left ventricular function and dimension. We have moved toward referring patients for surgery if they have significantly dilated ventricles (as compared with mean normal values) with documented progression in cavity dimension. This approach, of course, requires frequent, accurate echocardiographic studies. We have recommended yearly studies in many patients and as frequently as every 6 months in others. It is our hope that a more aggressive approach will serve to reduce the likelihood of irreversible left ventricular dysfunction.

We have felt that there are other patient-related criteria that have led us down a path of early aortic valve repair. There is ample evidence in the surgical and medical literature to support the fact that the therapeutic margin of safety in patients receiving oral anticoagulation for mechanical cardiac valves is at least in part related to the patient's own diligence in complying with dosages and therapeutic monitoring.[47] We have observed particular difficulty in managing anticoagulation in adolescent patients with mechanical valves. These patients may have great difficulty in accepting the necessity of lifelong medication and periodic blood tests. We have felt that the option of preserving the patient's native valve is very attractive in this group of individuals.

A case in point is that of a 15-year-old male referred to The Cleveland Clinic Foundation for evaluation and management of severe aortic insufficiency secondary to leaflet prolapse in a bicuspid aortic valve. This patient had been followed by a local cardiologist and had worsening aortic insufficiency and increasing left ventricular dimension. When first evaluated he had severe aortic insufficiency (4+ by echocardiography) and a left ventricular cavity dimension of 70 mm. The surgical options were reviewed in detail with the patient and his parents, including mechanical valve replacement, pulmonary autograft replacement, and aortic valve repair. Of particular importance to this young man was the fact that his greatest passion in life is skateboarding. He freely admitted that regardless of what valve he received, he would continue vigorous skateboarding, which is obviously a high-risk activity for a patient taking warfarin (Coumadin). We opted to proceed with aortic valve repair. This was accomplished with methods to be described later. Early postoperative echocardiographic studies demonstrated trivial aortic insufficiency and good left ventricular function. At the 1-year follow-up, the aortic insufficiency remains trivial, the patient's ventricular function is good, and his cavity dimension has decreased significantly. He continues to enjoy skateboarding.

## SURGICAL METHODS

### INTRAOPERATIVE MANAGEMENT

At the Cleveland Clinic Foundation, all patients undergoing an aortic valve repair have a preoperative transesophageal echocardiographic study performed in the operating room after the induction of general, endotracheal anesthesia. This study is invaluable in planning an operative strategy based on the morphologic features of the aortic valve. As noted previously, the nature of the aortic insufficiency, the morphology of the valve, the location of the regurgitation, the size of the aortic annulus, and an estimation of left ventricular function can all be determined by an experienced echocardiographer. This information is critical in assessing the feasibility of valve repair.

After standard median sternotomy and dissection, cardiopulmonary bypass is established by means of aortic and dual-staged right atrial cannulation. A coronary sinus retrograde perfusion catheter is used to achieve cardioplegic arrest, and the left atrium is vented via the right superior pulmonary vein.

The aortic valve is exposed via a transverse aortotomy. Heavy traction sutures of 2–0 silk are placed in the aortic wall immediately above the valve commissures. This facilitates exposure and assessment of the valve.

Following valve repair and resuscitation of the heart, the patient is weaned from cardiopulmonary bypass. At this time, the repair is carefully evaluated with transesophageal echocardiography. We would not accept an intraoperative result of anything worse than trivial (1+) aortic insufficiency. If necessary, the heart can be rearrested and additional maneuvers carried out as indicated.

## BICUSPID AORTIC VALVES

As noted previously, we have had the most success with repair of insufficient, congenitally bicuspid aortic valves. In such cases there is usually sufficient annulus size to allow valvuloplasty without causing stenosis. This is a critical point, however, and great care must be exercised to ensure an adequate annular dimension after repair.

After exposure of the valve, the two leaflets are examined. As noted previously, insufficiency is usually the result of prolapse of one leaflet. In this condition, this is most frequently the conjoined cusp. In viewing the prolapsing segment, it is usually apparent that the free edge of the conjoined leaflet is considerably longer than its counterpart. The prolapsing segment is often noted to be much thicker than adjacent normal segments of leaflet tissue. This thickened area occurs as the result of chronic regurgitant flow and is very useful in guiding the repair.

To achieve leaflet symmetry and remove the prolapsing segment, a triangular resection is undertaken. This resection is in the form of an equilateral triangle whose dimensions are determined by the length of excessive leaflet tissue with some allowance for the incorporation of tissue into the suture line. If present, the raphe is resected as well. After resection, the triangular defect is closed with a continuous, double-layered nonabsorbable multifilament suture. This closure represents a slight modification of our original technique in which we used interrupted sutures but found a late incidence of suture line dehiscence (Figs 4 to 6).

To achieve a greater area of leaflet coaptation or lunula, annular plication is frequently performed at both commissures. At this point, some degree of judgment has to be exercised to avoid excessive annular narrowing. The technique used was originally described by Cabrol and colleagues and employs the use of horizontal mattress sutures buttressed with Teflon felt placed through the annulus at each commissure.[37] The amount of leaflet coaptation is

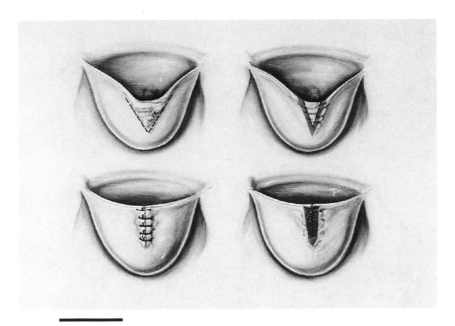

**FIGURE 4.**

Schematic representation of triangular cusp resection and repair. The area to be restricted is identified as the thickened segment of the prolapsing cusp. Our initial technique employed complete resection of the thickened area and closure with interrupted sutures (shown on the *left*). We have modified the technique to leave a small amount of tissue in the triangle to be incorporated into a continuous suture line.

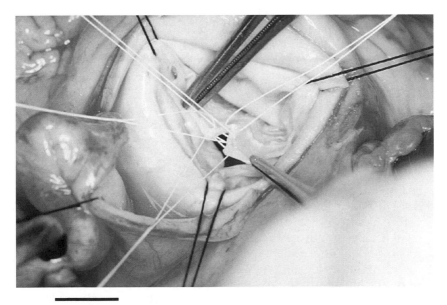

**FIGURE 5.**

Operative photograph of a cusp repair after triangular resection.

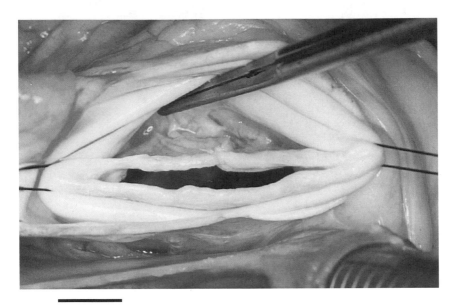

**FIGURE 6.**

Operative photograph documenting cusp symmetry after triangular resection and repair.

determined by the depth the sutures are placed in the aortic sinus. This governs the height of the interleaflet triangle and the amount of leaflet coaptation (Figs 7 and 8).

On rare occasions we have debrided the thickened leaflet in an attempt to achieve greater cusp mobility. Also, if there is an associated subaortic membrane, this is resected.

## TRICUSPID AORTIC VALVES

Tricuspid aortic valves with prolapse of a single cusp may also be amenable to repair. In such cases, the prolapsing cusp is elongated. In these situations a triangular resection is also performed to achieve cusp symmetry with leaflet repair as noted previously. Commissural plication sutures are then used to maximize leaflet coaptation (Fig 9, A and B).

We have limited attempts at repairing insufficient tricuspid valves because of prolapse to patients with a single prolapsing cusp. Patients with multiple prolapsing cusps are not amenable to repair and should undergo valve replacement.

As noted elsewhere, severe aortic insufficiency may develop in some young individuals after rheumatic fever as a result of thickening and infolding of the cusp edges. In such patients, the bellies of the cusps are often noted to be relatively normal. This finding

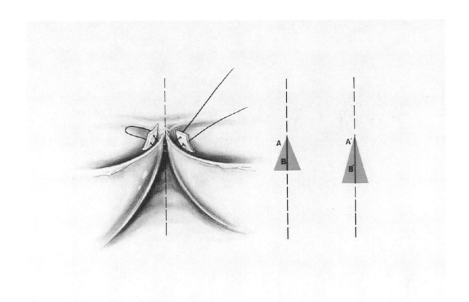

**FIGURE 7.**

Technique of commissuroplasty. Horizontal mattress sutures are placed through the base of the cusp (not to include the leaflet tissue). The sutures result in a taller, more narrow interleaflet triangle and thus a greater area of leaflet coaptation.

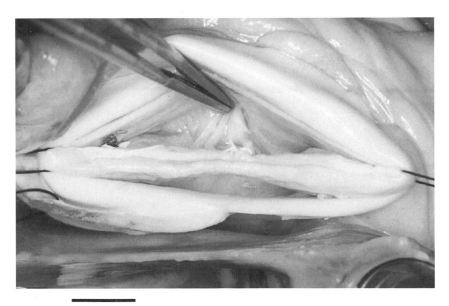

**FIGURE 8.**

Completed repair of a bicuspid valve with excellent leaflet coaptation.

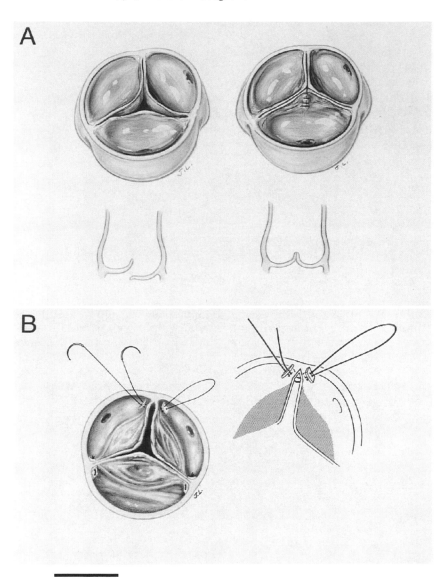

**FIGURE 9.**

The principles of repair may be applied to insufficient tricuspid valves. The prolapsing segment of an enlarged cusp is repaired by triangular resection **(A)**, and greater areas of leaflet coaptation area are achieved by subcommissural sutures **(B)**.

has led some to attempt valvuloplasty in these patients. Although we have no experience with this technique, we find the possibility intriguing. Duran and associates have recently published their experience with valvuloplasty using autologous pericardium in 49 such patients. Briefly, their method uses a strip of glutaraldehyde-treated autologous pericardium to augment the remaining cusp tissue after the abnormal portions have been removed. The early results are encouraging, but too preliminary to make firm recommendations. The reader is referred to this article for further details of the procedure.[48]

## PERFORATED/FENESTRATED VALVES

Fenestrations occurring at or near the commissures are frequently noted in otherwise normal aortic valves. Although usually of no hemodynamic consequence, these fenestrations occasionally enlarge enough to result in significant insufficiency. In such patients, resection of the fenestrated area with primary repair is adequate to correct the insufficiency (Fig 10).

An occasional patient with healed endocarditis will be left with a large cusp perforation, but otherwise normal valve. We have felt comfortable repairing the perforation in these instances with

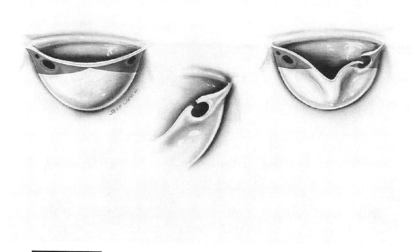

**FIGURE 10.**

Areas of cusp fenestration may be the source of significant insufficiency.

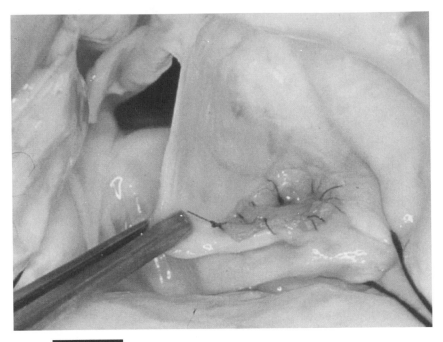

**FIGURE 11.**
Perforation from old endocarditis repaired with a pericardial patch.

autologous, untreated pericardial patches sewn in with a continuous polyproprylene suture (Fig 11).

## RESULTS

Our experience has been heavily weighted toward repair of insufficient bicuspid aortic valves. Since November 1988, we have performed valve repair in 88 such patients. The majority of individuals have been males (83), and the mean age at surgery has been 40
± 10 years. More than 75% of our patients have had isolated aortic valve repair procedures. Before surgery, 28% of the patients
were in New York Heart Association (NHYA) functional class I,
44% of the patients were class II, 25% were class III, and 2% were
class IV.

All patients in this group underwent a triangular leaflet resection as previously described. In addition, 97% of the patients underwent a commissural plication. Fifty percent of the patients had
a rudimentary raphe, which was resected.

We now have a mean follow-up in this group of patients approaching 30 months. To date, there have been no operative or late
deaths. The mean aortic occlusion time in this series has been 39

± 12 minutes. There have been no early or late strokes. Patients have not been anticoagulated postoperatively.

At last follow-up, 94% of the patients were in NYHA functional class I. Late postoperative echocardiographic studies have been performed in 58 patients, usually at the discretion of the referring cardiologist. At a mean of 16 ± 13 months postoperatively, the mean degree of aortic insufficiency is 0.89 ± 0.82. This compares very favorably with the preoperative value of 3.6 ± 0.6 ($P < .0001$).

Thus far, six patients have required reoperation from 4 days to 16 months after repair. By using the Kaplan-Meier method, freedom from aortic valve reoperation was calculated at 89.5% at 3 years (95% confidence limits, 81.3% to 97.7%). The causes of repair failure have included suture line dehiscence of the cusp repair in 3 patients at a time when we were using interrupted suture techniques.

An additional 20 patients have undergone repair of a tricuspid valve. Our follow-up is much more limited in this group of patients. Although encouraged, our impression is that valvuloplasty in this population may be less predictable than in patients with bicuspid valves.

## CONCLUSIONS

Our overall impression remains that in selected patients, aortic valvuloplasty is a viable therapeutic option. Successful applications of these techniques clearly requires very careful patient selection. Patients with insufficient bicuspid aortic valves are probably most amenable to this therapy.

The technical aspects of these operations are straightforward. The primary emphasis must be on careful preoperative assessment in selecting candidates and intraoperative evaluation of valve morphology via transesophageal echocardiography. The principles of proper functioning of the aortic valve can be used as guidelines to successful repair.

Although the long-term outcome of these patients is unknown, the short- and intermediate-term results remain encouraging. We are particularly enthusiastic about applying these methods to younger individuals in whom other options for valve replacement may be less satisfactory.

## REFERENCES

1. Taylor WJ, Thrower WB, Black H, et al: The surgical correction of aortic insufficiency by circumclusion. *J Thorac Cardiovasc Surg* 35:192–205, 1955.

2. Bailey CP, Bolton HE, Jamison WL, et al: Commissurotomy for rheumatic aortic stenosis. I. Surgery. *Circulation* 9:22–31, 1954.

3. Trusler GA, Moes CA, Kidd BS: Repair of ventricular septal defect with aortic insufficiency. *J Thorac Cardiovasc Surg* 66:394–403, 1973.

4. Spencer FC, Bahnson HT, Neill CA: The treatment of aortic regurgitation associated with a ventricular septal defect. *J Thorac Cardiovasc Surg* 43:222–233, 1962.

5. Ellis FH, Ongley PA, Kirlin JW: Ventricular septal defect with aortic valvular incompetence. Surgical consideration. *Circulation* 27:789–795, 1962.

6. Starr A, Edwards ML: Mitral replacement: Clinical experience with a ball-valve prosthesis. *Ann Surg* 154:726–740, 1961.

7. Barratt-Boyes, Roche AHG, Subramanyan R, et al: Long-term follow-up of patients with the antibiotic sterilized aortic homograft valve inserted freehand in the aortic position. *Circulation* 75:768–777, 1987.

8. Ross DN: Replacement of aortic and mitral valves by the pulmonary autograft. *Lancet* 2:956–958, 1967.

9. Matsuki O, Robles A, Gibbs S, et al: Long-term performance of 555 aortic homografts in the aortic position. *Ann Thorac Surg* 46:187–191, 1988.

10. Elkins RC, Santangelo K, Stelzer P, et al: Pulmonary autograft replacement of the aortic valve and evolution of technique. *J Card Surg* 7:108–116, 1992.

11. Lytle BW, Cosgrove DM, Taylor PC: Primary isolated aortic valve replacement. *J Thorac Cardiovasc Surg* 97:675–694, 1989.

12. Cohn LH, Allred EN, DeSesa VJ, et al: Early and late risk of aortic valve replacement. *J Thorac Cardiovasc Surg* 98:695–702, 1984.

13. Aranki S, Rizzo RJ, Couper GS, et al: Aortic valve replacement in the elderly: Effect of gender and coronary artery disease on operative mortality. *Circulation* 5(suppl 2):17–23, 1993.

14. Mitchell RS, Miller DS, Stinson EB, et al: Significant patient-related determinants of prosthetic valve performance. *J Thorac Cardiovasc Surg* 91:807–817, 1986.

15. Borkon AM, Soule LM, Baughman KL, et al: Comparative analysis of mechanical and bioprosthetic valves after aortic valve replacement. *J Thorac Cardiovasc Surg* 94:20–33, 1987.

16. Hartz RS, LoCicero J, Kucich V, et al: Comparative study of warfarin versus antiplatelet therapy in patients with a St. Jude Medical valve in the aortic position. *J Thorac Cardiovasc Surg* 92:684–690, 1986.

17. Cohn LH, Collins JJ, DiSesa VJ, et al: Fifteen year experience with 1678 Hancock bioprosthetic heart valve replacements. *Ann Thorac Surg* 210:435–443, 1989.

18. Jones EL, Weintraub WS, Craver JM, et al: Ten-year experience with the porcine valve: Interrelationship of valve survival and patient survival in 1,050 valve replacements. *Ann Thorac Surg* 49:370–384, 1990.

19. Yacoub MH, Rasmi NRH, Sundt TM, et al: Fourteen year experience with "Homovital" homografts for aortic valve replacement. *J Thorac Cardiovasc Surg,* 110:186–194, 1995.
20. Chon LH, DiSesa VJ, Collins JJ Jr: The Hancock modified orifice bioprosthetic valve: 1976–1988. *Ann Thorac Surg* 48:81–82, 1989.
21. Bloomfield P, Wheatley DJ, Prescott RJ, et al: Twelve year comparison of the Bjork-Shiley mechanical heart valve with porcine valve prosthesis. *N Engl J Med* 324:573–579, 1991.
22. Hammermeister KE, Sethi GK, Henderson WG, et al: A comparison of outcomes in men 11 years after heart valve replacement with a mechanical valve or bioprosthesis. *N Engl J Med* 328:489–496, 1993.
23. Albertucci M, Wong K, Petrou M, et al: The use of unstented homograft valves for aortic valve reoperations. Review of a twenty-three year experience. *J Thorac Cardiovasc Surg* 107:152–161, 1994.
24. Lytle BW, Cosgrove DM, Taylor PC, et al: Reoperations for valve surgery: Perioperative mortality and determinants of risk for 1000 patients, 1958–1984. *Ann Thorac Surg* 42:632–643, 1986.
25. Olson LJ, Subramanian R, Edwards WD: Surgical pathology of pure aortic insufficiency by Doppler color flow mapping. *J Am Coll Cardiol* 59:835–841, 1987.
26. Hallgrimsson J, Tulinius H: Chronic non-rheumatic aortic valvular disease: A population study based on autopsies. *J Chronic Dis* 32:355–361, 1979.
27. Mills P, Leech G, Davies M, et al: The natural history of a non-stenotic bicuspid aortic valve. *Br Heart J* 40:951–957, 1979.
28. Wilcox BR, Anderson RH: *Surgical Anatomy of the Heart.* New York, Raven Press, 1985.
29. Thubrikar M: *The Aortic Valve.* Boca Raton, Fla, CRC Press, 1990.
30. Thubrikar MJ, Aouad J, Nolan SP: Comparison of the in vivo and in vitro mechanical properties of aortic valve leaflets. *J Thorac Cardiovasc Surg* 92:29–36, 1986.
31. Thubrikar MJ, Bosher LP, Nolan SP: The mechanism of opening of the aortic valve. *J Thorac Cardiovasc Surg* 77:863–870, 1979.
32. Olson LJ, Subramanian, R, Edwards WD: Surgical pathology of pure aortic insufficiency: A study of 225 cases. *Mayo Clin Proc* 59:835–841, 1984.
33. Roberts WC, Morrow AG, McIntosh CL, et al: Congenitally bicuspid aortic valve causing severe, pure aortic regurgitation without superimposed infective endocarditis. *Am J Cardiol* 47:206–209, 1981.
34. David TE, Feindel CM: An aortic valve sparing operation for patients with aortic incompetence and aneurysm of the ascending aorta. *J Thorac Cardiovasc Surg* 103:617–622, 1992.
35. Bentall HH, DeBono A: A technique for complete replacement of the ascending aorta. *Thorax* 23:338–341, 1968.
36. Gott VL, Pyeritz RE, Magovern GJ, et al: Surgical treatment of aneurysms of the ascending aorta in the Marfan syndrome. *N Engl J Med* 314:1070–1074, 1986.

37. Cabrol C, Guiraudon G, Bertrand M, et al: Le traitement de l'insufficance aortique par l'annuloplastie aortique. *Arch Mal Coeur* 59:1305–1312, 1966.
38. Carpentier A: Cardiac valve surgery—the "French correction." *J Thorac Cardiovasc Surg* 86:323–337, 1983.
39. Ellis H, Ongley PA, Kirklin JW: Ventricular septal defect with aortic valvular incompetence. Surgical considerations. *Circulation* 27:789–792, 1963.
40. Keck EWD, Ongley PA, Kincaid DW, et al: Ventricular septal defect with aortic insufficiency: A clinical and hemodynamic study of 18 proved cases. *Circulation* 27:203–209, 1963.
41. Kirlin JE, Barratt-Boyes BD: *Aortic Valve Disease. Cardiac Surgery.* New York, Churchill Livingstone, 1993, pp 492–495.
42. Guiney TE, Davies MJ, Parker DJ, et al: The aetiology and course of isolated severe aortic regurgitation: A clinical, pathological and echocardiographic study. *Br Heart J* 58:358–364, 1987.
43. Duran C: Reconstructive techniques for rheumatic aortic valve disease. *J Card Surg* 3:23–28, 1988.
44. Perry GJ, Helmcke F, Navoa NC, et al: Evaluation of aortic insufficiency by Doppler color flow mapping. *J Am Coll Cardiol* 9:952–959, 1987.
45. Bonow RO, Rosing DR, McIntosh CL, et al: The natural history of asymptomatic patients with aortic regurgitation and normal left ventricular function. *Circulation* 68:509–517, 1983.
46. Scognamiglio R, Rahimtoola SH, Fasoli G, et al: Nifedipine in asymptomatic patients with severe aortic regurgitation and normal left ventricular function. *N Engl J Med* 331:689–694, 1994.
47. Horstkotte D, Schulte H, Bricks W, et al: Unexpected findings concerning thromboembolic complications and anticoagulation after complete 10 year follow up of patient with St. Jude medical prostheses. *J Heart Valve Dis* 2:291–301, 1993.
48. Duran C, Gallo R, Kumar N: Aortic valve replacement with autologous pericardium: Surgical technique. *J Card Surg* 10:1–9, 1995.

# Special Considerations in Cardiopulmonary Bypass*

### Joe R. Utley, M.D.

Division of Cardiac Surgery, Spartanburg Regional Medical Center, Spartanburg, South Carolina; Clinical Professor of Surgery, Medical University of South Carolina, Charleston, South Carolina; University of South Carolina School of Medicine, Columbia, South Carolina

### Glenn P. Gravlee, M.D.

Professor and Chairman, Department of Anesthesiology, Allegheny Campus, Medical College of Pennsylvania and Hahnemann University, Pittsburgh, Pennsylvania

---

C ardiopulmonary bypass (CPB) has been conducted with hemodilution and hypothermia for many years. Many of the techniques and methods of performing CPB have been the subjects of recent intense study and scrutiny. Continuous pressure to improve outcomes and reduce costs has simultaneously led to the application of new technologies and re-evaluation of standard CPB technologies. As a result, new equipment, methods, and approaches have been applied to almost every aspect of CPB. The most difficult challenge imposed by these efforts has been to separate the morbidity induced by CPB from that caused by the patient's disease and the cardiac procedure itself.

## TEMPERATURE OF PERFUSION

Varying degrees of hypothermia have been used by virtually every cardiac surgeon. Most surgeons employ moderate (28 to 32° C) or mild (33 to 35° C) hypothermia, although some have routinely selected more profound levels (22 to 27° C). A common practice has been to let the temperature drift downward toward room temperature during bypass without specifically using the heat exchanger for cooling. Recently some surgeons have routinely combined normothermic systemic perfusion with normothermic retrograde blood cardioplegia. Even with "normothermic" perfusion the ac-

---

*This work was supported by the Cardiothoracic Research and Education Foundation.

tual temperature has varied with the technique. Heat losses from the patient and the bypass circuit are so large that in order to maintain the patient's temperature at 37° C, the water bath temperature must be set at 38 or 38.5° C. With the water bath of the heat exchanger set at 37° C, the patient's temperature will still drift downward to induce mild hypothermia (33 to 35° C).

Several factors have caused surgeons and perfusionists to reexamine perfusion temperatures. With greater degrees of hypothermia, the rewarming period contributes importantly to cost and morbidity. Because operating room time is so expensive, shortening the rewarming time may significantly decrease cost. Complement activation and presumably other surface activation phenomena are much more pronounced at warmer temperatures than at cooler ones.[1] Rewarming constitutes the majority of the perfusion time other than the aortic crossclamp period. This non-clamp perfusion time strongly predicts morbidity and mortality after coronary bypass grafting.[2] Many reasons have been cited in the prevailing trend to perform operations at warmer temperatures, but there are some potential drawbacks to this technique.

Normothermic CPB is associated with vasodilation and with greater release of catecholamines, steroids, insulin, glucagon, cytokines, tumor necrosis factor, interleukin-6, and interleukin-1β. Normothermia also appears to accelerate the activation of clotting factors and the fibrinolytic system, although platelet function may be better preserved. No significant difference in postoperative bleeding has been observed.[3-12]

Truly normothermic perfusion, which requires continuous active warming, carries a greater risk of associated neurologic injury.[3] Oxygen desaturation of the jugular venous blood signifies insufficient brain oxygen supply relative to demand. Jugular venous blood desaturation is more common and severe with normothermic than with hypothermic perfusion. A possible explanation for the increased risk of brain injury is that normothermia or slight hyperthermia renders the brain more vulnerable to injury from the microemboli showers that are commonly produced toward the end of CPB and while it is terminated. This does not, however, explain the greater risk of neurologic injury with continuous normothermia than with return to normothermia by rewarming at the end of CPB. Traditional methods of temperature monitoring do not accurately reflect brain temperature, which undoubtedly contributes importantly to the problem. Mild degrees of perfusion hypothermia (33 to 35° C) are less likely than truly normothermic perfusion to be associated with neurologic injury.[13]

## HEMATOCRIT

The safety of hemodilution during CPB and the risk of blood transfusion have caused surgeons and anesthesiologists to push the limits of hemodilution during and after CPB. Blood salvage techniques enable the surgeon to perform cardiac operations with very little loss of the patient's red cell mass. Many surgeons have experienced situations in which perfusion at a low hematocrit seemed satisfactory until termination of CPB. In some patients, CPB cannot be terminated with stable hemodynamics until the hematocrit is raised by blood transfusion. Our clinical observations show that the hematocrit is less than 20% in virtually all patients in whom this situation develops. The concept has therefore developed that very low hematocrit levels (15% to 20%) may be safe during CPB but may be inadequate when CPB is terminated.[14]

The indication for transfusion during CPB is almost always low hematocrit rather than hypovolemia or bleeding. Recent analysis of mortality and morbidity figures after coronary artery bypass grafting at Spartanburg Regional Medical Center shows that the strongest predictor of a poor outcome is transfusion in the operating room.[15] This may be an important reason for the greater risk of coronary artery bypass grafting in women and the elderly. Preoperative strategies to preserve and restore red cell mass need to be evaluated to determine whether they might decrease the risk of coronary artery bypass grafting in patients with small red cell mass from anemia or small body size.[15] Although the need for transfusion for a low hematocrit during CPB is associated with an increased risk, a direct cause-and-effect relationship has not been proved.

## ANTICOAGULATION: HEPARIN AND PROTAMINE MANAGEMENT

### HEPARIN MANAGEMENT

We believe that many cardiac surgical teams continue to place patients at undue risk for excessive postoperative bleeding by overdosing them with heparin and protamine. Evidence is accumulating that overdosing with heparin increases postoperative bleeding, although the mechanism remains unclear. Some work suggests that heparin rebound accounts for this occurrence, whereas another paper suggests that excessive heparin doses produce sustained platelet dysfunction that does not respond to protamine.[16-18] One recent paper suggests that larger doses of heparin may be slightly protective (or at least unharmful) when

CPB durations tend to be as long as 2.5 hours.[19] Factors predisposing to unnecessary heparin overdosing may include a propensity among manufacturers of heparin monitoring devices and oxygenators to make precautionary recommendations without supporting data. In some cases, these recommendations are self-serving, in essence exploiting fears among cardiac surgeons, anesthesiologists, and perfusionists about inadequate anticoagulation.

Several misconceptions can lead to heparin overdosing. First, there is a misconception about the utility of the activated coagulation time (ACT) during CPB[20, 21] that is based on the correct observation that the relationship between blood heparin concentration and ACT changes during CPB. The primary reason for this change is that hypothermia and hemodilution legitimately enhance anticoagulation, thus prolonging the ACT. Some believe that this altered relationship mandates the more expensive use of heparin concentration monitoring, which invariably increases heparin doses substantially. Since the primary concern should be that anticoagulation is adequate, we should continue to use the ACT to monitor anticoagulation adequacy while recognizing that rewarming from 28° C to normothermia may decrease the ACT by 50 to 100 seconds. For those conducting CPB at temperatures of 32° C or higher, this effect will be proportionately reduced.

Another frequently expressed concern is that ACTs become unreliable when they exceed 600 seconds. The ACT is a somewhat imprecise test by nature, and its imprecision increases as its value increases. So what? It matters not if the same patient produces paired ACT values of 650 and 750 seconds. The bottom line is that any patient with ACTs exceeding 600 seconds is fully anticoagulated (possibly overanticoagulated). One does not need to confirm this by measuring blood heparin concentrations. This may not be the case in the presence of aprotinin when celite is the coagulation activator for the ACT, in which case some have recommended maintaining celite ACTs over 750 seconds; kaolin-activated ACTs need not be altered during aprotinin use.

Another factor leading to unnecessary heparin overdosing is undue fear of inadequate anticoagulation in patients receiving heparin infusions preoperatively. Although these patients do manifest heparin resistance when compared with patients not receiving heparin preoperatively, in most patients this effect is relatively mild.[22, 23] Consequently, these patients need not routinely receive higher heparin doses before CPB. When patients such as these show heparin resistance, some clinicians panic by administering either fresh-frozen plasma or enormous heparin doses to achieve unnecessarily high ACT values such as 500 seconds. If the ACT exceeds 300 seconds and the CPB priming solution has a heparin concentration greater than 2 USP units/mL (e.g., 5,000 units for most prime volumes less than 2,000 mL), just begin CPB and get on with the surgery.

Table 1 shows our opinions about appropriate, cost-effective heparin dosing and monitoring for CPB. One other cost-cutting consideration is the heparin tissue source. In the United States, either effective pharmaceutical marketing or outdated fears have sustained the more costly use of bovine lung heparin for cardiac surgery, although data supporting this need are sparse, dated, and probably clinically irrelevant. In Europe, porcine mucosal heparin is commonly used for cardiac surgery. The same should be true in the United States.

The impact of biocompatible surfaces on heparin management continues to evolve. Some reports suggest that reduced ACTs (200 to 300 seconds) can be safely used with heparin-coated surfaces,[24, 25] whereas anecdotal reports of clotting in areas of stasis (e.g., the left atrium while rewarming after mitral valve replacement) cause concern.[26] This area needs further study since some European reports suggest reduced intraoperative and postoperative blood losses if lower ACTs are combined with heparin-coated surfaces.

---

**TABLE 1.**
Recommended Heparin Dosing and Monitoring
for Cardiopulmonary Bypass

1. Draw blood for baseline ACT* after the surgical incision (ACT reaches its lowest point at that time).
2. Give heparin (porcine mucosal or bovine lung), 300 units/kg, before cannulation.
3. Add heparin, 2 units/mL (5,000 units for adults), to CPB prime.
4. Wait 3 minutes, measure ACT. Go on CPB if ACT > 300 sec.
5. If blood temperature < 30° C, maintain ACT > 400 sec. If blood temperature < 24° C, maintain ACT > 500 sec.
6. If ACT < 300 sec after heparin administration of > 900 units/kg, give fresh frozen plasma, 2 units, or antithrombin III concentrate, 1,000–2,000 units.

*ACT = activated clotting time; CPB = cardiopulmonary bypass.

## PROTAMINE MANAGEMENT

Some centers continue to practice as though the following statement axiomatically applies: "if a little protamine is good, then more is better." We believe that this practice constitutes a myth perpetuated from the early days of cardiac surgery, when it was not uncommon to use protamine-to-heparin dose ratios as high as 2:1 (2 mg of protamine per 100 units of heparin). In the first place, one need not neutralize heparin that has been metabolized or excreted, so neutralizing the total dose of heparin administered is unnecessary. In the second place, it only takes 1.1 to 1.2 mg of protamine to neutralize 100 units of heparin. Although some believe that excessive doses of protamine create a free protamine "reserve supply" to accommodate potential heparin rebound, the pharmacoki-

---

**TABLE 2.**

Protamine Dosing Recommendations

1. If ACT*-guided heparin dosing has been used as suggested in Table 1, assume that the plasma heparin concentration is less than that present before initiating bypass.
2. Give 2–3 mg of protamine for each 100 units of heparin administered before CPB. Ignore supplemental doses given during CPB and placed in the priming solution.
3. Check the ACT. If the ACT is within 10 sec of the postincision baseline ACT, proceed to sternal closure unless coagulopathy is present. If coagulopathy exists, give an additional 25 mg of protamine because a small amount of unneutralized heparin may remain even if the ACT has returned to baseline.
4. Add 20 mg of protamine for each 500 mL of unprocessed blood infused from the residual contents of the extracorporeal circuit after completing separation from CPB and initial protamine administration. If the reinfused blood has been concentrated and washed (e.g., Cell Saver), do not give additional protamine because the heparin has been washed out.
5. If heparin rebound is suspected, give protamine, 25 mg once an hour. If this seems insufficient, repeat the ACT and give an additional 25 mg if the ACT still exceeds the postneutralization baseline by more than 10 sec. If still in doubt, use a laboratory test that reliably identifies heparin presence (not ACT unless protamine corrected).

---

*ACT = activated clotting time; CPB = cardiopulmonary bypass.

netics of free protamine in human plasma remain ill-defined, but there is little doubt that even moderate protamine excess in animals depresses platelet function and the platelet count.[27] Since some combination of thrombocytopenia and depressed platelet function constitutes the predominant cause of post-CPB coagulopathy, why exacerbate this problem by perpetuating myths about protamine dosing? Substantial protamine excess depresses plasma coagulation as well.[28]

Human studies suggest increased postoperative bleeding when neutralization ratios exceeding 1:1 (for the total heparin dose) are used.[29, 30] This area needs further investigation in humans to better define the magnitude of protamine overdose required to significantly increase bleeding, but why worry? Just give sufficient protamine to neutralize the circulating heparin and accept the possibility that a small additional dose may be required later for heparin rebound. There is also a possibility, as yet unproven or controversial in humans, that protamine unbound to heparin predisposes to adverse hemodynamic or pulmonary reactions—another potential reason for avoiding excessive protamine doses.[31] Table 2 shows our suggestions about protamine dosing for adults.

# PHARMACOPROPHYLAXIS AGAINST POST–CARDIOPULMONARY BYPASS BLEEDING

## ANTIFIBRINOLYTIC DRUGS

The use of antifibrinolytic agents to prevent post-CPB coagulopathy has shown recent explosive growth. Most centers appear to be using ε-aminocaproic acid (EACA) frequently or routinely for this purpose, whereas others choose aprotinin or nothing. What is the correct strategy? Abundant literature now confirms that both synthetic (EACA and tranexamic acid) and naturally occurring (aprotinin) antifibrinolytics decrease blood loss and transfusion requirements in cardiac surgery.[32] Aprotinin may be more efficacious than the synthetic antifibrinolytics,[33] but this will not be clarified until more prospective direct comparisons are performed. In some studies, transfusion outcomes have been biased toward favorable outcomes for aprotinin by using unnecessarily high transfusion triggers (e.g., requiring hemoglobin concentrations greater than 10 g/dL after CPB regardless of patient stability). Clearly, aminocaproic acid is effective and very inexpensive, but one could argue that aprotinin is more appropriate for patients who are at a very high risk for excessive postoperative bleeding. Regardless of the antifibrinolytic agent chosen, high doses administered before and during bypass are necessary for optimal protection, which probably occurs principally by protecting platelets from the adverse effects of CPB. One study suggests that aprotinin effectively neutralizes the adverse bleeding outcomes induced by unnecessarily high heparin doses, whereas a similar outcome results from traditionally conservative heparin doses alone. Recent scientific abstracts suggest the possibility that low-risk patients undergoing primary coronary revascularization do not benefit from prophylactic antifibrinolytic therapy in the presence of relatively short CPB times and low transfusion triggers.[34, 35]

Controversy also surrounds the issue of potentially increased risks for perioperative thrombotic events in patients receiving antifibrinolytic drugs. This issue has been closely evaluated for aprotinin as part of the drug approval investigations preceding its release by the Food and Drug Administration. Although the possibility remains that there is a small adverse effect on coronary graft patency, it appears unlikely that this effect is clinically significant for aprotinin or for the synthetic antifibrinolytics. Case reports suggest the occurrence of electrocardiographic ST-segment changes[36] or clot formation on pulmonary artery catheters when antifibrinolytic agents are administered before heparin administration. Consequently, it appears increasingly common to withhold antifibrinolytic agents until heparin has been given. We agree with this practice but wonder whether this will reduce the effectiveness of the prophylaxis in view of inconsistent aprotinin efficacy when it is placed only in the CPB priming solution. Is it possible that systemic administration of high-dose aprotinin 5 minutes before initiating CPB is effective while similar doses placed in the CPB priming solution are not? Most studies showing efficacy have initiated aprotinin before or at surgical incision, yet we are now concerned about pre-CPB thrombotic risks when selecting this strategy with any of the antifibrinolytic agents. Table 3 shows our current recommendations for antifibrinolytic prophylaxis.

## DESMOPRESSIN
Although the initial report was highly favorable, numerous subsequent studies have failed to support prophylactic administration of desmopressin after heparin neutralization. Some studies do suggest a strong possibility that it may be a useful treatment for post-CPB coagulopathy attributable to platelet dysfunction.[37, 38] We believe that desmopressin constitutes reasonable treatment for post-CPB coagulopathy while awaiting the preparation of platelet concentrates or other blood components, but we do not recommend

**TABLE 3.**
Antifibrinolytic Prophylaxis in Cardiac Surgery With
Cardiopulmonary Bypass

1. Use aminocaproic acid for most cases. Loading dose, 150 mg/kg after anticoagulation with heparin; maintenance, 10 mg/kg/hr. Discontinue when heparin is neutralized.
2. Use high-dose aprotinin for very high-risk cases if the patient has not been previously exposed to it. Load with 2 million KIU for most adults, 2 million KIU in CPB* prime, and give 500,000 KIU/hr until heparin is neutralized. Manage heparin and ACT as indicated in Table 1, but use kaolin (not Celite) as the ACT activator.
3. Avoid aprotinin for deep hypothermic circulatory arrest cases until further studies have established its safety in that situation.

*CPB = cardiopulmonary bypass; ACT = activated clotting time.

its prophylactic use. Since desmopressin vasodilates arterioles, its administration may require the concomitant administration of an α-adrenergic agonist.

## TECHNOLOGY

Continued improvement in the technology of CPB promises to decrease the damaging effect of the intervention. Membrane oxygenators, arterial filters, centrifugal pumps, white blood cell filters, and heparin-bonded circuits have been introduced as methods of reducing the injurious effects of CPB.

Membrane oxygenators are widely used and have been shown to be advantageous by limiting the activation of blood components. Activation of complement and white cells and release of the products of activation processes are less frequent with membrane than with bubble oxygenators. Membrane oxygenators that have a closed, collapsible venous reservoir are less likely to pass large amounts of air and result in air embolization.[39-47]

Centrifugal pumps are becoming increasingly popular for routine CPB. Centrifugal pumps are less injurious to blood cellular and plasma components than are occlusive roller pumps. The potential for massive air embolization is less with centrifugal pumps than with roller pumps because of their diminished capacity to pump large amounts of air. The safety of centrifugal pumps has been questioned because of their propensity to backflow if the amount of revolutions per minute is diminished or stopped.[48-51]

Even more controversial is the use of heparin-bonded circuits. Heparin-bonded circuits hold some promise of decreasing the activation of blood components by the foreign surface, diminishing coagulopathy and bleeding, and simplifying anticoagulant management.[52-56]

A review of the information concerning improvement in patient outcome with the use of advanced technology in CPB does not reveal convincing data that outcomes are improved.[57] Technology that has been examined includes pulsatile flow, centrifugal pumps, membrane oxygenators, arterial line filtration, leukocyte-depleting filters, ultrafiltration, heparin-coated circuits, and in-line blood gas monitoring. Why are improved outcomes so difficult to prove? Many studies are imperfectly designed with historical and nonrandomized controls, failure of double blinding, and inappropriate use of statistics. With the relatively low frequency of adverse outcome events, a very large sample size is necessary to have a high level of confidence that a significant difference has not been missed. Proof of improved outcomes is becoming increasingly important as pressure for reducing costs intensifies. Proof that technological advances are beneficial to patients may be most easily demonstrated with high-risk operations.

The pressure to decrease costs has resulted in suppliers marketing plus surgeons and perfusionists purchasing packaged bypass systems that include tubing, oxygenator, filters, pump heads, reservoirs, and cardioplegia system from one supplier. In the future, the pressures of cost containment may lead to the development of a low-cost package of low-technology components that can be safely used for low-risk operations. Such a system may include a bubble oxygenator, roller pump, and minimal or no filtration. In many parts of the world the demand for cardiac surgery so far exceeds the supply that packaging and pricing strategies to reduce cost may significantly increase the volume of cases.

## REFERENCES

1. Moore FD, Warner KG, Assousa S, et al: The effects of complement activation during cardiopulmonary bypass. *Ann Surg* 208:95–103, 1988.
2. Utley JR, Morgan MS, Johnson HD, et al: Correlates of total perfusion time, clamp time, and non-clamp perfusion time in coronary bypass surgery. *Perfusion* 4:205–211, 1989.
3. Martin TD, Craver JM, Gott JP, et al: Perspective, randomized trial of retrograde warm blood cardioplegia: Myocardial benefit and neurologic threat. *Ann Thorac Surg* 57:298–304, 1994.

4. Naylor DC, Lichtenstein SV, Fremes SE, et al: Randomized trial of normothermic versus hypothermic coronary bypass surgery. *Lancet* 343:559–563, 1994.
5. Wong BI, McLean RF, Naylor CD, et al: Central-nervous-system dysfunction after warm or hypothermic cardiopulmonary bypass. *Lancet* 339:1383–1384, 1992.
6. Cook DJ, Oliver WC Jr, Orszulak TA, et al: A prospective, randomized comparison of cerebral venous oxygen saturation during normothermic and hypothermic cardiopulmonary bypass. *J Thorac Cardiovasc Surg* 107:1020–1029, 1994.
7. Menasche P, Haydar S, Peynet J, et al: A potential mechanism of vasodilation after warm heart surgery. The temperature-dependent release of cytokines. *J Thorac Cardiovasc Surg* 107:292–299, 1994.
8. Singh AK, Feng WC, Bert AA, et al: Warm body, cold heart: Myocardial revascularization in 2383 consecutive patients. *J Cardiovasc Surg* 334:415–421, 1993.
9. Lehot JJ, Vilolard J, Piriz H, et al: Hemodynamic and hormonal responses to hypothermic and normothermic cbp. *J Cardiothorac Vasc Anesth* 6:132–139, 1992.
10. Lehot JJ, Piriz H, Villard J, et al: Glucose homeostasis. Comparison between hypothermic and normothermic cardiopulmonary bypass. *Chest* 102:106–111, 1992.
11. Croughwell ND, Frasco P, Blumenthal JA, et al: Warming during cardiopulmonary bypass is associated with jugular bulb desaturation. *Ann Thorac Surg* 53:827–832, 1992.
12. Christakis GT, Koch JP, Demmar KA, et al: A randomized study of the systemic effects of warm heart surgery. *Ann Thorac Surg* 54:449–459, 1992.
13. Guyton RA: Normothermic cardiopulmonary bypass. Presented at the 15th Annual San Diego Cardiothoracic Surgery Symposium, Feb 23, 1995.
14. Cooper JR Jr, Slogoff S: Hemodilution and priming solutions for cardiopulmonary bypass, in Gravlee GP, Davis RF, Utley JR (eds): *Cardiopulmonary Bypass: Principles and Practice*. Baltimore, Williams & Wilkins, 1993, pp 93–123.
15. Utley JR, Wilde EF, Leyland SA, et al: Intraoperative blood transfusion as major factor for coronary artery bypass grafting in women. *Ann Thorac Surg* 60:570–575, 1995.
16. Gravlee GP, Haddon WS, Rothberger HK, et al: Heparin dosing and monitoring for cardiopulmonary bypass: A comparison of techniques with measurement of subclinical plasma coagulation. *J Thorac Cardiovasc Surg* 99:518–527, 1990.
17. Gravlee GP, Rogers AT, Dudas LM, et al: Heparin management protocol for cardiopulmonary bypass influences postoperative heparin rebound but not bleeding. *Anesthesiology* 76:393–401, 1992.
18. Boldt J, Schindler E, Osmer CH, et al: Influence of different antico-

agulation regimens on platelet function during cardiac surgery. *Br J Anaesth* 73:639–644, 1994.

19. Despotis GJ, Joist JH, Hogue CW, et al: The impact of heparin concentration and activated clotting time monitoring on blood conservation: A prospective, randomized evaluation in patients undergoing cardiac operation. *J Thorac Cardiovasc Surg* 110:46–54, 1995.

20. Culliford AT, Gitel SN, Starr N, et al: Lack of correlation between activated clotting time and plasma heparin during cardiopulmonary bypass. *Ann Surg* 193:105–111, 1981.

21. Cohen, EJ, Cameriengo IJ, Dearing JP: Activated clotting times and cardiopulmonary bypass I: The effect of hemodilution and hypothermia upon activated clotting time. *J Extracorp Technol* 12:130–141, 1980.

22. Dietrich W, Spannagl M, Schramm W, et al: Richter JA. The influence of preoperative anticoagulation on heparin response during cardiopulmonary bypass. *J Thorac Cardiovasc Surg* 102:505–514, 1991.

23. Staples MH, Dunton RF, Karlson KJ, et al: Heparin resistance after preoperative heparin therapy or intraaortic balloon pumping. *Ann Thorac Surg* 57:1211–1216, 1994.

24. von Segesser LK, Weiss BM, Garcia E, et al: Reduced blood loss and transfusion requirements with low systemic heparinization: Preliminary clinical results in coronary artery revascularization. *Eur J Cardiothorac Surg* 4:639–643, 1990.

25. von Segesser LK, Weiss BM, Garcia E, et al: Reduction and elimination of systemic heparinization during cardiopulmonary bypass. *J Thorac Cardiovasc Surg* 103:790–799.

26. Cheung AT, Levin SK, Weiss SJ, et al: Intracardiac thrombus: A risk of incomplete anticoagulation for cardiac operations. *Ann Thorac Surg* 58:541–542, 1994.

27. Velders AJ, Wildevuur ChRH: Platelet damage by protamine and the protective effect of prostacyclin: An experimental study in dogs. *Ann Thorac Surg* 42:168–171, 1986.

28. Dutton DA, Hothersall AP, McLaren AD, et al: Protamine titration after cardiopulmonary bypass. *Anaesthesia* 38:264–268, 1983.

29. Moriau M, Masure R, Hurlet A, et al: Haemostasis disorders in open heart surgery with extracorporeal circulation: Importance of the platelet function and the heparin neutralization. *Vox Sang* 32:41–51, 1977.

30. Guffin AV, Dunbar RW, Kaplan JA, et al: Successful use of a reduced dose of protamine after cardiopulmonary bypass. *Anesth Analg* 55:110–113, 1976.

31. Tan F, Jackman H, Skidgel RA, et al: Protamine inhibits plasma carboxypeptidase N, the inactivator of anaphylatoxins and kinins. *Anesthesiology* 70:267–275, 1989.

32. Horrow JC: Management of coagulopathy associated with cardiopulmonary bypass, in Gravlee GP, Davis RF, Utley JR (eds): *Cardiopulmonary Bypass: Principles and Practice*. Baltimore, Williams & Wilkins 1993, pp 436–466.

33. Fremes SF, Wong BI, Lee E, et al: Metaanalysis of prophylactic drug treatment in the prevention of postoperative bleeding. *Ann Thorac Surg* 58:1580–1588, 1994.
34. Ralley FE, DeVarennes B, Robitaille M: Comparison of aprotinin vs. tranexamic acid vs. placebo on blood loss for elective CABG surgery: Are they necessary? *Anesth Analg* 80(suppl 4):137, 1995.
35. Hardy JF, Belisle S, Robitaille D, et al: Prophylactic E-aminocaproic acid or tranexamic acid do not decrease bleeding and transfusions after primary CABG. *Anesth Analg* 80(suppl 4):135, 1995.
36. Robblee J: Graft occlusion following administration of tranexamic acid. *Anesth Analg* 80(suppl 4):141.
37. Mongan PD, Hosking MP: The role of desmopressin acetate in patients undergoing coronary artery bypass surgery: A controlled clinical trial with thromboelastographic risk stratification. *Anesthesiology* 77:38–46, 1992.
38. Despotis, GJ, Grishaber JE, Goodnough LT: The effect of an intraoperative treatment algorithm on physicians' transfusion practice in cardiac surgery. *Transfusion* 34:290–296, 1994.
39. Boonstra PW, Vermeulen FEE, Leusink JA, et al: Hematological advantage of a membrane oxygenator over a bubble oxygenator in long perfusions. *Ann Thorac Surg* 41:297–300, 1986.
40. Clark RE, Beauchamp RA, Magrath RA, et al: Intracardiac thrombus: A risk of incomplete anticoagulation for cardiac operations. *Ann Thorac Surg* 58:541–542, 1994.
41. Dancy CM, Townsend ER, Boylett A, et al: Pulmonary dysfunction associated with cardiopulmonary bypass: A comparison of bubble and membrane oxygenators. *Circulation* 64(suppl 2):11–54, 1981.
42. Hessel EA II, Johnson DD, Ivey TD, et al: Membrane versus bubble oxygenator for cardiac operations: A prospective randomized study. *J Thorac Cardiovasc Surg* 1:111–122, 1980.
43. Reeve WG, Ingram SM, Smith DC: Respiratory function after cardiopulmonary bypass: A comparison of bubble and membrane oxygenators. *J Cardiothorac Vasc Anesth* 8:502–508, 1994.
44. Sade RM, Bartles DM, Dearing JP, et al: A prospective randomized study of membrane versus bubble oxygenators in children. *Ann Thorac Surg* 29:502–511, 1980.
45. Utley JR, Leyland SA, Johnson HD, et al: Correlation of preoperative factors, severity of disease, type of oxygenator and perfusion times with mortality and morbidity of coronary disease. *Perfusion* 6:15–22, 1991.
46. van den Dungen JJAM, Karliczek GF, Brenken U, et al: Clinical study of blood trauma during perfusion with membrane and bubble oxygenators. *J Thorac Cardiovasc Surg* 83:108–116, 1982.
47. van Oeveren W, Kazatchkine MD, Descamps-Latscha B, et al: Deleterious effects of cbp: A prospective study of bubble versus membrane oxygenation. *J Thorac Cardiovasc Surg* 89:888–889, 1985.

48. Kolff J, Ankley RN, Wurzel D, et al: Centrifugal pump failures. To be presented at the 33rd Annual Meeting of the Pennsylvania Association for Thoracic Surgery, Sept 15, 1995.

49. Driessen JJ, Freansen G, Rondelez L, et al: Comparison of the standard roller pump and a pulsatile centrifugal pump for extracorporeal circulation during routine coronary artery bypass grafting. *Perfusion* 6:303–311, 1991.

50. Jakob HG, Hafner G, Iverson S, et al: Reoperation and the centrifugal pump. *Eur J Cardiothorac Surg* 6 (suppl 1):59–63, 1992.

51. Jakob HG, Hafner G, Thelemann C, et al: Routine extracorporeal circulation with centrifugal versus roller pump. *ASAIO Trans* 37:487–489, 1991.

52. Boonstra PW, Gu YJ, Akkerman A, et al: Heparin coating of an extracorporeal circuit partly improves hemostasis after cardiopulmonary bypass. *J Thorac Cardiovasc Surg* 107:289–292, 1994.

53. Edmunds LH: Surface-bound heparin: Panacea or peril? *Ann Thorac Surg* 58:285–286, 1994.

54. Gravlee GP: Heparin-coated cardiopulmonary bypass circuits. *J Cardiothorac Vasc Anesth* 8:213–222, 1994.

55. Sellevold OFM, Berg TM, Rein KA, et al: Heparin-coated circuit during cardiopulmonary bypass: A clinical study using closed circuit, centrifugal pump and reduced heparinization. *Acta Anaesthesiol Scand* 38:372–379, 1994.

56. Wagner WR, Johnson PC, Thompson KA, et al: Heparin-coated cardiopulmonary bypass circuits: Hemostatic alterations and postoperative blood loss. *Ann Thorac Surg* 58:734–741, 1994.

57. Hessel EA II: Debate: Technical advances in CPB equipment: Does benefit justify cost? Presented at the 15th Annual Meeting of the San Diego Cardiothoracic Surgery Symposium, Feb 24, 1995.

# Surgical Implications in Hearts With Isomeric Atrial Appendages

**Hideki Uemura, M.D.**

Department of Cardiovascular Surgery, National Cardiovascular Center, Osaka, Japan; Department of Paediatrics, National Heart and Lung Institute, London, England

**Robert H. Anderson, M.D.**

Professor, Department of Paediatrics, National Heart and Lung Institute, London, England

**Toshikatsu Yagihara, M.D.**

Department of Cardiovascular Surgery, National Cardiovascular Center, Osaka, Japan

S ince the reports regarding multiple spleens by Abernethy in 1793[1] and absence of the spleen by Martin in 1826,[2] the coexistence of abnormal splenic status and congenital heart defects has long been stressed. Because of these historical precedents, it became customary to describe and distinguish these cardiac malformations in terms of "asplenia" and "polysplenia" syndromes. Van Mierop and Wiglesworth[3] and Moller et al.,[4] while retaining those titles, also emphasized the important tendency in these syndromes toward isomerism of the thoracic organs. Indeed, as long ago as 1962, Van Mierop and Wiglesworth[3] established that in asplenia, not only was the bronchial tree isomeric, but so were the atrial appendages and the sinus nodes. In spite of these observations, some groups of investigators and clinicians still seem unable or unwilling to divorce themselves from the splenic monster. They still insist on usage of the terms "asplenia" and "polysplenia" when describing cardiac malformations. Recognition of these syndromes is undoubtedly helpful for clinicians to visualize those congenital visceral abnormalities that might be present in any given patient and, importantly, could affect the prognosis. Splenic status, however, is obviously not an ideal device with which to describe precisely the cardiac malformations. During open heart surgery, for instance, knowledge of splenic agenesis in a patient does not provide direct information for an effective construction of the intra-atrial pathway. Instead, it is precise identification of the structural features within the heart itself that, to us, provides the most appropriate guide for surgical treatment of each patient. As we will show in this chapter, recognition of an isomeric arrangement of the atrial appendages is all that is needed for optimal analysis of visceral heterotaxy. Nonetheless, detailed and correct morphologic diagnosis in any individual patient is needed not only for the atrial components but also for all the other anatomic features of the heart. Analysis in this fashion then shows that there are more generalized structural differences between the groups of hearts with isomerism of the morphologically right appendages, those with left isomerism, and those with the usual atrial arrangement. This strongly suggests that identification of isomeric atrial appendages is of significance for surgeons so as to select optimal surgical strategies.

In fact, the number of surgical procedures is increasing markedly in patients with isomeric atrial appendages or those with visceral heterotaxy. In the setting of right isomerism, maintenance of proper pulmonary circulation is the paramout initial requirement, this requiring frequent creation of systemic-to-pulmonary shunts because of the presence of pulmonary stenosis or atresia or requiring the repair of pulmonary venous obstructions because of totally anomalous pulmonary venous connections. In patients with left isomerism, in contrast, it is reconstruction of the obstructed outflow tract of the morphologically left ventricle or repair of aortic coarctation that is more likely to be a crucial part of staged operations. Nowadays, however, not only these palliative procedures but also definitive correction of the circulation, either through anatomic biventricular repair or definitive functional procedures, are more likely to be used. Although several groups have described successful anatomic repair in the setting of right isomerism,[5-7] the number of such repairs remains small, probably reflecting the high incidence of univentricular atrioventricular connections and the unusual ventricular architecture found in such patients. When biventricular repair is contraindicated, a Fontan-type operation becomes the alternative "corrective" procedure of choice. Some have constructed an unobstructed pathway from the inferior caval vein to the pulmonary arteries in the fashion of a total cavopulmonary connection.[8, 9] These maneuvers certainly seem to have improved surgical outcomes, particularly in the short term, and have overcome many of the difficulties in intra-atrial rerouting of blood produced by the abnormal veno-atrial connections that are an integral part of these syndromes. Furthermore, in recent years regurgitation across the atrioventricular valves has been clinically recognized as one of the major risk factors for poor surgical outcome after the Fontan-type procedure in the short and long term.[10, 11] This problem is particularly pertinent in the setting of patients with isomeric atrial appendages. When a total bypass operation of the right side of the heart is contraindicated by major risk factors, a total cavopulmonary shunt for hearts with interruption of the inferior caval vein, originally proposed by Kawashima and his colleagues,[12] a bidirectional Glenn procedure,[13-15] or a hemi-Fontan procedure[16] can be alternative procedures providing "semidefinitive" surgery or can be part of a staged approach aimed at eventually producing a complete Fontan circulation. From our clinical experience, it has been regurgitation of the atrioventricular valve, frequently associated with ventricular dysfunction, that has emerged as one of the factors most likely to demand attention after such partial right heart bypass operations.

In this chapter, therefore, we begin by emphasizing those features that permit surgical recognition of isomerism. We then highlight the hazardous features of atrioventricular valvar regurgitation and ventricular dysfunction in patients with isomeric atrial appendages, as well as the suitability of such patients for anatomic biventricular repair. Toward this purpose, we first describe the surgical experience of definitive and semidefinitive surgery in our series of patients with isomeric atrial appendages who had been referred to the National Cardiovascular Center in Osaka, Japan. We then interpret these clinical results in the light of morphologic findings in a large series of autopsied specimens. We have also used our morphologic findings to comment on the continuing debate concerning the salient features of the heart in patients with so-called visceral heterotaxy.[17, 18]

## RECOGNITION OF ISOMERIC ARRANGEMENT OF THE ATRIAL APPENDAGES

Although precise morphologic distinction of the atrial appendages occasionally remains problematic when viewed externally, we have now found that the most characteristic marker of a morphologically right appendage is the extent of the pectinate muscles around the vestibule of the atrioventricular junctions. Thus, pectinate muscles meeting at the crux are the rule in hearts with right

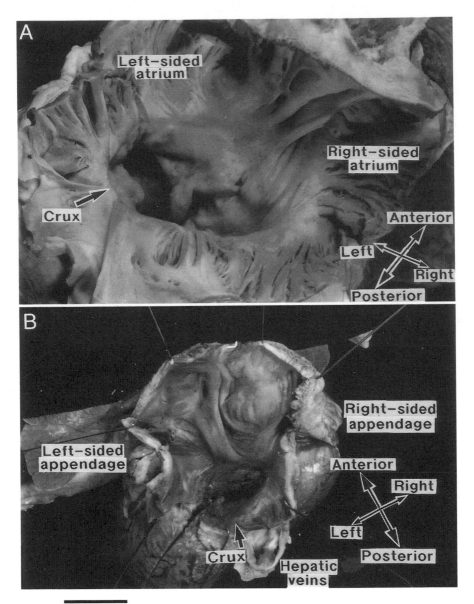

**FIGURE 1.**

**A,** pectinate muscles in hearts with isomerism of morphologically right appendages, with the posterior extensions of the muscles meeting at the crux of the heart. **B,** in hearts with isomeric left appendages, the pectinate muscles did not reach the crux bilaterally, and a confluent area was left between the smooth component of the atrium and the vestibule of the atrioventricular junction.

isomerism (Fig 1,A). In contrast, in those with left isomerism, the pectinate muscles do not extend posteriorly, and a smooth internal surface is left on both sides between the vestibule of the atrioventricular junction and the venous component of the atrial wall (Fig 1,B). In our own series of 182 autopsied specimens exhibiting visceral heterotaxy, the shape of appendages, their junctions with the rest of the atrial component, and the unequivocal presence of

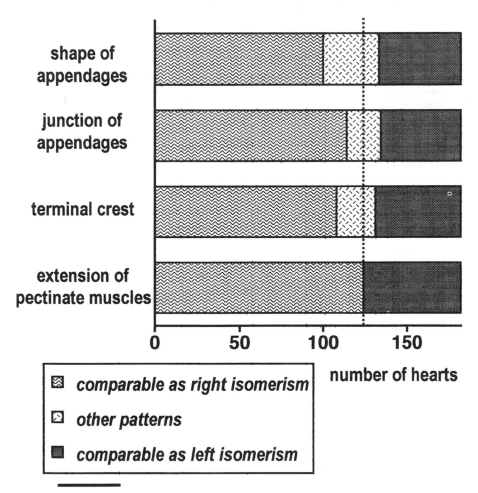

**shape of appendages**

**junction of appendages**

**terminal crest**

**extension of pectinate muscles**

0    50    100    150

**number of hearts**

☒ *comparable as right isomerism*

◨ *other patterns*

■ *comparable as left isomerism*

**FIGURE 2.**
External and internal features of atrial appendages. Shapes and junctions of atrial appendages can occasionally be of an intermediate pattern. The bilateral presence or absence of pectinate muscles at the crux of the heart, in contrast, has proved to be an unequivocal landmark for determining the arrangement of the atrial appendages.

a terminal crest were good indicators for determining the isomeric arrangement of atrial appendages, but not absolute criteria. In contrast, the characteristic extension of the pectinate muscles, either bilaterally present or bilaterally absent, proved to be an unequivocal marker (Fig 2). Pulmonary lobation, bronchial pattern, and splenic status were concordant with the arrangement of the isomeric atrial appendages in 71.7%, 90.9%, and 79.9% of the hearts, respectively (Table 1).

These arrangements, namely, the presence or absence of pectinate muscles at the crux of the heart, are readily determined at the time of surgery. They could also, we predict, be diagnosed preop-

---

**TABLE 1.**

Isomeric Atrial Appendages, Pulmonary Arrangement, and Splenic Status

| | **Bronchial Pattern** | | | |
| | **Bilaterally Short** | **Bilaterally Long** | **Others** | **Unknown** |
|---|---|---|---|---|
| Right isomerism | 98* | 0 | 14 | 12 |
| Left isomerism | 0 | 51 | 1 | 6 |
| Incidence of concordance | | 90.9% | | |

| | **Pulmonary Lobes** | | | |
| | **Bilaterally Trilobes** | **Bilaterally Bilobes** | **Others** | **Unknown** |
|---|---|---|---|---|
| Right isomerism | 79 | 2 | 31 | 12 |
| Left isomerism | 2 | 40 | 12 | 4 |
| Incidence of concordance | | 71.7% | | |

| | **Splenic Status** | | | |
| | **Absent** | **Present (Multiple)** | **Present (Solitary)** | **Unknown** |
|---|---|---|---|---|
| Right isomerism | 70 | 4 | 17 | 33 |
| Left isomerism | 2 | 37 | 4 | 15 |
| Incidence of concordance | | 79.9% | | |

*Values are numbers of cases.

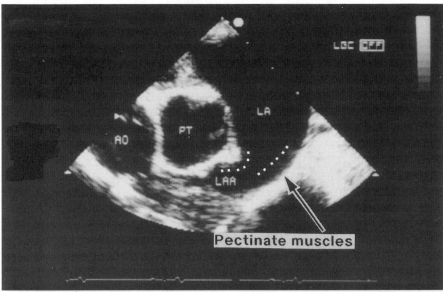

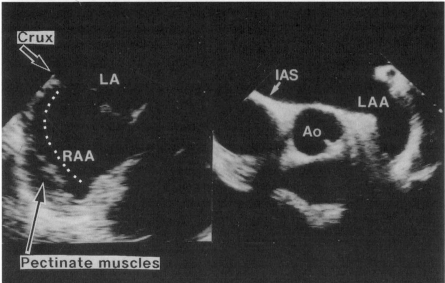

**FIGURE 3.**

Transesophageal echocardiography demonstrates not only the shape of atrial appendages but also the degree of extension of the pectinate muscles. These pictures were taken from patients with the usual atrial arrangement. *LA* = left atrium; *RAA* = right atrial appendage; *IAS* = interatrial septum; *LAA* = left atrial appendage; *Ao* = aorta; *PT* = pulmonary trunk.

eratively by using transesophageal echocardiography (Fig 3). Because the hemodynamic environment can influence and change the shape of cardiac structures,[17] it is the morphology itself at the junctions of the appendages that we have used unequivocally to identify the presence of isomeric appendages.

## DEFINITIVE AND SEMIDEFINITIVE SURGERY IN PATIENTS WITH ISOMERISM OF THE ATRIAL APPENDAGES

During the past 10 years, 55 patients with isomerism of the morphologically right appendages and 37 with left isomerism underwent definitive or semidefinitive surgery at the National Cardiovascular Center in Osaka, Japan. Among the group of patients with isomerism of the morphologically right atrial appendages, anatomic biventricular repair could be achieved in only 3 patients (5%), whereas functional biventricular repair in which the morphologically right ventricle was used to support the systemic circulation and the left ventricle was used for the pulmonary circulation was achieved in a further 2 (4%) patients. A Fontan-type procedure was performed in 40 patients, 2 having had a previous bidirectional Glenn procedure. The remaining 10 patients undergoing a bidirectional Glenn procedure have not proceeded to further surgical treatment either because of the presence of undesirable risk factors compromising a successful Fontan-type procedure or because of their subsequent death. As for the group of patients with left isomerism, anatomic biventricular repair was the most common procedure, being employed in 25 patients (68%). A total cavopulmonary connection (a Fontan-type procedure) was chosen in 7, including 4 in whom the procedure was achieved after the creation of so-called total cavopulmonary shunts (by means of bidirectional cavopulmonary anastomosis). Five patients undergoing such partial right heart bypass operations have not proceeded to further definitive surgery. Our preference is to strive for anatomic biventricular repair whenever possible while recognizing the potential superiority of a situation in which the morphologically left ventricle ejects blood for the systemic circulation in conjunction with support of the pulmonary circulation by ventricular contractions. The proportion of anatomic biventricular repairs accomplished in our series of patients, therefore, illustrates the well-known fact that the underlying morphology of patients with right as opposed to left isomerism is less suitable for anatomic definitive repair.

## ANATOMIC BIVENTRICULAR REPAIR

Anatomic biventricular repair was extensive and complicated in three patients with right isomerism. The first patient, a 6-year-old girl, underwent repair of a totally anomalous pulmonary venous connection concomitant with atrial septation. Ventricular maneuvers included intraventricular rerouting using a baffle after enlargement of the ventricular septal defect and creation of a pathway from the right ventricle to the pulmonary arteries via an external conduit. The second patient, a 5-year-old male, simultaneously underwent repair of a totally anomalous pulmonary venous connection, division of a common atrioventricular valve, intraventricular rerouting of blood, atrial septation, and reconstruction of the right ventricular outflow tract with a patch. The third patient, a 6-year-old boy, underwent repair of a totally anomalous pulmonary venous connection, division of a common atrioventricular valve, intraventricular rerouting, intra-atrial rerouting via a Mustard procedure, and construction of the right ventricular outflow tract with an external conduit. To divide a common atrioventricular valve concomitant with intraventricular rerouting, the maneuver described by Pacifico and his colleagues[6] was employed. The first and the third patients had undergone previous construction of systemic-to-pulmonary shunts. All these procedures were successful in the short term, but the third patient died 2 months after surgery of anaphylactic shock induced by blood transfusion. The other two patients are doing well, although the second patient shows recurrence of regurgitation across the morphologically left atrioventricular valve. Their long-term outcome remains a matter of concern.

Similar extensive surgery needed to accomplish anatomic biventricular repair was carried out in seven patients with left isomerism. Intra-atrial rerouting combined with intraventricular rerouting and use of an external conduit was performed in four patients 3 to 9 years of age. One patient died of multiple organ failure. The other three patients underwent division of a common atrioventricular valve and atrial septation concomitant with either repair of the tetralogy of Fallot (in one patient) or intraventricular rerouting after enlargement of the ventricular septal defect and reconstruction of the right ventricular outflow tract with a patch, the ages at surgery being 3, 2, and 3 years, respectively. Among these three patients, one died of ventricular dysfunction, probably due to injury to the septal branch of one of the coronary arteries during myocardial resection for enlargement of the ventricular septal defect. All except the patient with coexisting tetralogy of Fallot had undergone previous construction of systemic-to-pulmonary shunts.

Less complicated definitive procedures were done in the remaining patients with left isomerism. Atrial septation was the surgical procedure in four patients without atrioventricular septal defects. In another six with atrioventricular septal defects and separate right and left atrioventricular valves, atrial septation as well as plasty of the inlet valves was achieved at ages ranging from 4 months to 4 years, with one patient undergoing simultaneous repair of coarctation of the aorta. Intra-atrial rerouting of blood by means of a Mustard procedure was necessary in four patients 6 to 18 months of age; systemic venous drainage was rerouted into the morphologically right ventricle and pulmonary venous drainage into the morphologically left ventricle. In one of them, simultaneous repair of the coarcted aorta was also performed. Three patients with an atrioventricular septal defect and a common atrioventricular valve underwent atrial and ventricular septations with a "two-patch" technique at the ages of 4 months, 7 months, and 3 years, respectively. Previous banding of the pulmonary trunk had been done in two patients. These procedures were successfully accomplished with no operative mortality in the 16 patients. The last patient, a 13-year-old boy with the tetralogy of Fallot, later died after the corrective surgery as a result of left ventricular dysfunction and pulmonary hypertension.

In total, the operative mortality for anatomic biventricular repair was 14% (4 of 28). Of the survivors, 1 additional death has occurred in a patient with left isomerism who underwent repair of an atrioventricular septal defect. The cause was regurgitation of the morphologically left atrioventricular valve. Reoperations were necessary nonetheless, in another 4 patients for plasty (in 1) or replacement (in 3) of the morphologically left atrioventricular valve after the initial surgical repair of the atrioventricular septal defect. In addition, 1 patient with right isomerism has recurrently shown moderate-to-severe regurgitation of the left component of the common atrioventricular valve, and further surgical treatment may be required in the near future. The morbidity concerning atrioventricular insufficiency is therefore 25% in the long term after definitive surgery. This incidence is statistically higher ($P < .01$, chi-square test) than results in our patients with the usual atrial arrangement who are undergoing repair of atrioventricular septal defects. During the same 10-year period, 109 patients survived such intracardiac repair, with 2 late deaths and 5 reoperations required for regurgitation across the morphologically left atrioventricular valve

(6%). It is therefore crucial to note that recurrence or development of atrioventricular valvar regurgitation is one of the frequent postoperative features of anatomic repair in patients with isomerism and a common atrioventricular valve.

## FUNCTIONAL BIVENTRICULAR REPAIR

Functional biventricular repair in which the morphologically right ventricle supports the systemic circulation and the left ventricle supports the pulmonary circulation was performed in two patients with right isomerism. The first, a 6-year-old boy, underwent atrial septation, closure of a ventricular septal defect via the arterial trunks, and connection of the morphologically left ventricle to the pulmonary arteries with an external conduit. This patient survived the operation but died suddenly 1½ years later, probably because of arrhythmia. This functional biventricular repair was performed 9 years ago, before we first performed a double-switch operation in 1987. If the patient had been seen today, we would have attempted to achieve anatomic repair. At the age of 5 years, the other patient underwent intra-atrial rerouting as well as replacement of the morphologically right component of the common atrioventricular valve, the inserted prosthetic valve functioning as an inlet valve for the systemic morphologically right ventricle. This patient remains asymptomatic and is doing well. Thus far, there has been no sign of ventricular dysfunction. This patient was considered unsuitable for switching at either the arterial or ventricular levels because of the presence of pulmonary stenosis and the absence of a ventricular septal defect.

## TOTAL RIGHT HEART BYPASS OPERATION (FONTAN-TYPE PROCEDURE)

The majority of patients with right isomerism were morphologically unsuitable for biventricular repair. Accordingly, a Fontan-type procedure was the definitive option chosen in 40 patients. Additionally, in the group of patients with left isomerism, 7 patients have undergone this type of functional repair when the intracardiac abnormalities made biventricular repair less than attractive. The ages at surgery ranged from 1.5 to 16.5 (8.5 ± 3.4) years. We opted for total cavopulmonary connection by means of either intra-atrial grafting with a polytetrafluoroethylene (Gore-Tex) tube or intra-atrial rerouting with an equine pericardial (Xenomedica) baffle. In 14 patients with right isomerism (30% of all patients), concomitant repair of the atrioventricular valves was added in an attempt to minimize postoperative deleterious regurgitation. The surgery involved plasty of either the valvar leaflets or their annulus in 13 patients and replacement of the valve in 1.

Operative mortality, including all operative and hospital deaths, was 23% (11 of 47). Early death related to residual regurgitation of the common atrioventricular valve was seen in 2. Pulmonary complications were the major cause of death in 3, circulatory insufficiency led to multiple organ failure in 4, and intractable arrhythmia was the problem in one. The remaining patient, a 4-year-old girl, died of severe peritonitis secondary to intestinal perforation. In spite of the fact that the patient was extubated and doing well, this accident occurred after she had taken several meals. The problem could well be related to the malrotation of the gut known to accompany visceral heterotaxy. Since this experience, we have applied, as preoperative intestinal preparation, a low-fiber diet and oral administration of kanamycin, like the pretreatment usually employed for gut surgery.

Of 36 operative survivors, late death has occurred in 2 patients with right isomerism. One child, a 3-year-old girl at the time of the Fontan-type procedure, died suddenly 8 months after the operation. Respiratory trouble was suspected. In the other, a 7-year-old girl, the postoperative course had been uneventful. No additional surgery for the atrioventricular valve had been deemed necessary at the time of her definitive operation. Nonetheless, 4 months after total cavopulmonary connection, the child began to suffer from progressive regurgitation of the common atrioventricular valve along with ventricular dysfunction. These features were more prominent across the morphologically left component than on the morphologically right side. Six months after the initial operation, replacement of the common atrioventricular valve became necessary, but the patient did not survive the surgery. We were unable to establish the precise cause of the progressive valvar regurgitation and irreversible ventricular dysfunction. The only finding at the time of reoperation, as well as at postmortem, was the presence of organized thrombus around the intra-atrial baffle used for connecting the inferior caval vein to the pulmonary arteries.

Recurrence of moderate-to-severe regurgitation of the atrioventricular valve has been recognized in 4 of 34 long-term survivors, with 3 having coexisting ventricular dysfunction. Isolated ventricular dysfunction of unknown origin has been seen in another 2. All of these patients have isomerism of the morphologically right appendages. Morbidity related to either valvar regurgitation or ventricular dysfunction has therefore thus far occurred in 22% (8 of 36) of our patients, including the patient who underwent simultaneous replacement of the atrioventricular valve at the time of total cavopulmonary connection.

## PARTIAL BYPASS OPERATION OF THE RIGHT SIDE OF THE HEART BY BIDIRECTIONAL CAVOPULMONARY ANASTOMOSIS

We have used a bidirectional Glenn procedure, or a total cavopulmonary shunt, as semidefinitive surgery or part of a staged procedure aimed eventually at total cavopulmonary connection for patients considered to be at too great a risk for successful achievement of total right heart bypass. These surgical procedures have been undertaken in 21 patients over our 10-year study period, valvar plasty being concomitantly performed in 7 (33%). Six of these 21 patients (29%) have subsequently been successfully converted to the Fontan-type circulation. Operative death after this partial right heart bypass occurred in 2 patients (10%) as a result of residual moderate regurgitation of the common atrioventricular valve exacerbated by supraventricular tachyarrhythmias and multiple organ failure triggered by gastric bleeding. Late death has been seen in 6 (29%). The major causes have been valvar regurgitation along with ventricular dysfunction in 2 and pneumonia, pulmonary venous obstruction after repair of a totally anomalous pulmonary venous connection, development of a pulmonary arteriovenous fistula, and sudden death, probably caused by an arrhythmia, in 1 each. The clinical course of the 2 patients dying of progressive valvar regurgitation with ventricular dysfunction was similar to that described earlier for the patient after total cavopulmonary connection, although valvar replacement was not attempted. The time between the bidirectional cavopulmonary anastomosis and late death was 4 and 16 months, respectively. Among 7 long-term survivors who have not undergone a Fontan-type procedure, reoperation for plasty of the atrioventricular valve was done in 1 patient, whereas another patient had previously undergone replacement of the common atrioventricular valve before the bidirectional Glenn procedure. Morbidity related to valvar regurgitation in the long term has therefore been 31% in this group of 13 patients surviving a bidirectional cavopulmonary anastomosis, excluding those who proceeded to a total right heart bypass operation. All cases of hazardous regurgitation were seen in patients with right isomerism.

## MORPHOLOGIC STUDY

To provide morphologic information relative to these problems identified at surgery, we have investigated a series of autopsied specimens from the collections of four institutions, namely, the National and Heart Lung Institute in London; Children's Hospital of Pittsburgh, Pennsylvania; the National Cardiovascular Center in Suita, Osaka, Japan; and the Royal Liverpool Children's Hospital in Liverpool, England. The total number of hearts examined was 182, 124 with right and 58 with left isomerism.

## CONNECTIONS BETWEEN VEINS, ATRIA, VENTRICLES, AND ARTERIAL TRUNKS

It is the abnormal combination of veno-atrial, atrioventricular, and ventriculo-arterial connections that makes surgical procedures more complicated when attempting anatomic biventricular repair. In particular, the patterns of systemic and pulmonary veno-atrial

**TABLE 2.**
Incidence of Abnormalities

| Abnormality | Right Isomerism* | Left Isomerism* |
|---|---|---|
| Abnormalities in systemic venous drainage | | |
| Superior caval vein | 4+ | 4+ |
| Inferior caval vein | 3+ | 5+ |
| Hepatic veins | 2+ | 4+ |
| Coronary sinus | 5+ | 3+ |
| Abnormalities in pulmonary venous drainage | | |
| Some or all via the extracardiac channel | 3+ | 1+ |
| All directly to the atrial chambers | 3+ | 3+ |
| Overall abnormalities in veno-atrial connections | 5+ | 5+ |
| Atrial septal defect | 5+ | 5+ |
| Atrioventricular connections | | |
| Biventricular and ambiguous | 3+ | 3+ |
| Double inlet | 3+ | 2+ |
| Absent right or left | 1+ | 2+ |
| Atrioventricular valves | | |
| Common orifice | 5+ | 3+ |
| Separate orifices (atrioventricular septal defect) | 1+ | 1+ |
| A solitary valve (absent atrioventricular connection) | 1+ | 2+ |
| Tricuspid and mitral valves | 1+ | 2+ |

| | | |
|---|---|---|
| Ventricular topology | | |
| Right-hand pattern† | 3+ | 4+ |
| Left-hand pattern‡ | 3+ | 2+ |
| Indeterminate | 1+ | 1+ |
| Ventricular septal defect | 5+ | 4+ |
| Ventriculo-arterial connections | | |
| Concordant | 1+ | 3+ |
| Discordant | 1+ | 1+ |
| Double outlet from the ventricle§ | 3+ | 3+ |
| Absent pulmonary outlet | 3+ | 1+ |
| Absent aortic outlet | 1+ | 1+ |
| Subarterial obstruction | | |
| Subpulmonary | 4+ | 3+ |
| Subaortic | 1+ | 3+ |
| Dual | 1+ | 1+ |

*+1 = 0% to 10%; +2 = 11% to 25%; +3 = 26% to 75%; +4 = 76% to 90%; +5 = 91% to 100%. Ranges are approximate.
†Including a dominant morphologically left ventricle (mLV) with a rudimentary and incomplete morphologically right ventricle (mRV) to the right and a dominant mRV with a rudimentary and incomplete mLV to the left.
‡Including a dominant mLV with a rudimentary and incomplete mRV to the left and a dominant mRV with a rudimentary and incomplete mLV to the right.
§Double outlet from the mRV or a solitary and indeterminate ventricle.

---

connections are almost always abnormal in the setting of isomerism of atrial appendages[19] (Table 2).

## VENO-ATRIAL CONNECTIONS

### Systemic Venous Drainage

In the group of hearts with right isomerism, bilateral superior caval veins were connected to the atrial roofs in 50% of the hearts, whereas a unilateral structure was joined to the right-sided (28%) or left-sided (22%) atrium in the remainder. The inferior caval vein was a solitary and uninterrupted structure connected to the right-sided (50%) or left-sided (50%) atrium, but part of the hepatic drainage was directed independently to the atrial cavities in 23% of the hearts (Fig 4). The pattern in which all the systemic veins joined directly to one atrium via superior and inferior caval veins was seen in only 29% of the hearts.

In hearts with left isomerism, dual superior caval veins were seen in 62%, either connected bilaterally to the atrial roofs (38%) or with one draining via the coronary sinus (24%). A solitary superior caval vein was connected to the right-sided atrium in 22%

and to the left-sided chamber in 16% of the hearts. The inferior caval vein was interrupted and drained via the azygous vein in 78% of the hearts, being right-sided in 37% and left-sided in 41%. In these hearts, the hepatic veins were connected directly to the atrium through a single orifice in three fifths, whereas two or more orifices for hepatic venous drainage were found in the remaining two fifths. When the inferior caval vein was uninterrupted, all hepatic veins joined the caval vein in 57%, with part of the drainage occurring via independent pathways in 43% (Fig 4). Overall, all systemic veins drained into one atrium in 40% of the hearts, but a

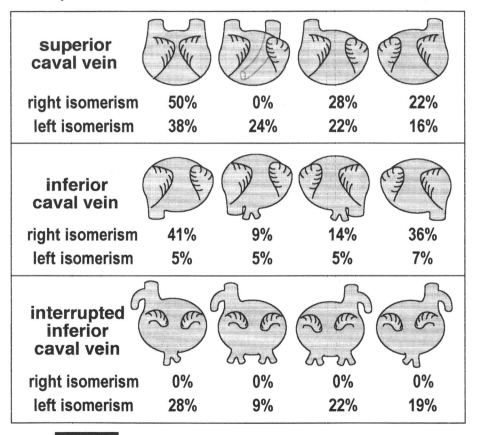

**FIGURE 4.**

Connections of the systemic veins to the atrial chambers. Overall, systemic venous drainage into one atrial chamber as seen in the normal hearts occured in only 29% and 5% of the cases with right and left isomerism of the atrial appendages, respectively.

pattern comparable to that seen in a normal heart was found in only 5% of this group of hearts.

Recognition of these morphologic patterns is of clinical importance not only for designing appropriate intra-atrial surgical maneuvers but also for establishing effective cardiopulmonary bypass.

## Pulmonary Venous Drainage

In 48% of the hearts with right isomerism, all pulmonary veins drained through a confluent pathway to an extracardiac site. Such extracardiac connection of the pulmonary veins was not seen in hearts with left isomerism. In left isomerism, bilateral connections, with the left pulmonary veins connected to the left-sided atrium and the right veins connected to the right-sided one, were the most common pattern (60%), whereas unilateral connection of all four veins to one atrial chamber was seen in the remaining two fifths of cases. Direct connection of all pulmonary veins to the atria was also seen in 42% of the hearts with right isomerism. The cardiac connection in right isomerism, however, was markedly different from the pattern seen in those with left isomerism. In right isomerism, the four pulmonary veins were almost always connected by way of a confluence with fibrous rather than muscular walls, as if forming a common pulmonary venous chamber. In the remainder of the cases with right isomerism (10%), one or two lobes of the lung drained independently without joining to the confluence between the other pulmonary veins.

When planning surgical repair of hearts with abnormal pulmonary venous connections, it is necessary to recognize the location of all the pulmonary venous connections in hearts with left isomerism. In right isomerism, it is the potential obstruction between the fibrous pulmonary venous confluence and the atrial chamber that is paramount, along with the precise pattern of extracardiac connections. If these points are ignored, residual lesions could persist or else pulmonary venous obstruction might develop and deleteriously affect the long-term outcome.

## Overall Pattern of Venous Drainage

Drainage of all the systemic veins into one atrium with connection of the pulmonary veins to the other atrium was seen in 13 hearts with isomeric right appendages (10%) and in 8 of those with isomeric left appendages (14%). If ventricular morphology is also taken into consideration for possible anatomic biventricular repair, simple procedures such as closure of an atrial septal defect would have proved to be the option of choice in only 1 of our postmortem specimens with right isomerism (1%) and in 4 with left isomerism (7%).

## ATRIOVENTRICULAR CONNECTIONS

Biventricular and ambiguous atrioventricular connections were seen in 56 hearts with right isomerism (45%) and in 43 with left isomerism (74%). Among these, an atrioventricular septum was present along with morphologically tricuspid and mitral valves in 4 and 7 hearts, respectively. In the rest of the hearts, the atrioventricular connections had a univentricular pattern: a dominant morphologically right ventricle in the presence of a rudimentary and incomplete morphologically left ventricle in 31% (of the hearts with right isomerism) and 14% (of those with left isomerism), a dominant morphologically left ventricle with a rudimentary and incomplete morphologically right ventricle in 20% (right isomerism) and 7% (left isomerism), and a solitary and indeterminate ventricle in 4% (right isomerism) and 5% (left isomerism).

## VENTRICULO-ARTERIAL CONNECTIONS

Concordant ventriculo-arterial connections were seen in only 4% of the hearts with right isomerism but accounted for 45% of those with left isomerism. Discordant connections were present in 9% and 2%, respectively. A double outlet from the morphologically right ventricle or from the solitary and indeterminate ventricle was relatively frequent in the settings of both right (35%) and left (43%) isomerism. A single outlet via the aorta with pulmonary atresia was the most common connection in hearts with right isomerism (50%) but was much less common in those with left isomerism (7%). Its partner, a single outlet via the pulmonary trunk with aortic atresia, was seen in 2% and 3%, respectively. In one exceptional case with right isomerism, a common arterial trunk arose from the morphologically right ventricle. Overall, obstructive lesions to the pulmonary arteries caused by either pulmonary atresia or stenosis were very frequent in the setting of right isomerism (85%) but less frequent in hearts with left isomerism (40%). Obstruction to the ascending aorta and/or at the aortic arch was more often seen in left isomerism (43%) than in right isomerism (11%).

## MORPHOLOGIC FEATURES OF A COMMON ATRIOVENTRICULAR VALVE AND ITS TENSION APPARATUS

When considering possible anatomic substrates for atrioventricular valvar regurgitation, three major features can be considered: the annular attachments, the structure of the leaflets, and the arrangement of the subvalvar tension apparatus. It is well known from surgical experience with the mitral valve[20-22] that structural abnormalities in the papillary muscles can also influence ventricular function. Furthermore, impaired ventricular function might be induced by inappropriate coronary circulation, as well as by coexisting abnormalities in ventricular mass. With all these features in mind, several morphologic investigations were performed on this large number of specimens.

## Annular Attachment of a Common Atrioventricular Valve

The annular attachment of a common atrioventricular valve was examined in 83 hearts, 60 with isomerism of the morphologically right and 23 with isomerism of the morphologically left atrial appendages. Only 5 hearts were found with a planar annular hinge point (6%) (Fig 5,A). All the others showed a nonplanar undulating arrangement. If the posterior half of the valvar attachment was taken as a reference point, the anterior part of the annulus markedly deviated in a superior fashion in 31 cases (37%), the distance between the reference to the point of greatest deviation horizontally being more than 10% of the circumferential length of the valvar annulus (Fig 5,B). The mean value for this distance in all cases was 8.5% ± 5.4% of the circumference. Further investigation revealed that the ratio of this distance, when compared with the anteroposterior diameter of the atrioventricular orifice, was greater in hearts with biventricular and ambiguous atrioventricular connections (0.36 ± 0.23) than in those with a double inlet to the dominant ventricle (0.24 ± 0.17) ($P < .01$, $t$-test). No significant differences were found when the hearts were analyzed according to the type of isomeric arrangement of the appendages or the presence or absence of fibrous continuity between the leaflets of the common atrioventricular valve and the arterial valves. On the basis of this finding, we recommend that the precise features of the annular structure of the common atrioventricular valves be examined preoperatively by cross-sectional or three-dimensional echocardiography so as to optimally plan effective annuloplasty or establish better surgical strategies.

## Arrangement of Papillary Muscles Within the Morphologically Left Ventricle

For this investigation, we studied all specimens with atrioventricular septal defects having a common atrioventricular valve and biventricular (either ambiguous or concordant) atrioventricular connections: 35 with isomerism of the morphologically right atrial appendages and 23 with left isomerism. As a control group, 33

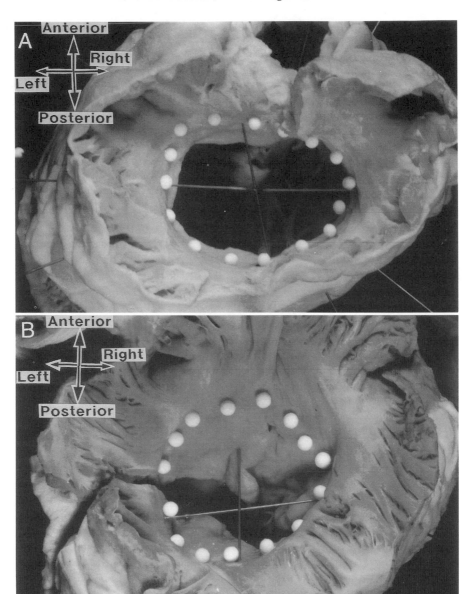

**FIGURE 5.**

**A,** planar attachment of a common atrioventricular valve. Annular attachments of atrioventricular valvar leaflets were planar in several hearts. The *cross* represents the planar level and the *white pinheads* mark the valvar insertion. **B,** a nonplanar undulating arrangement was much more frequent, the anterior part of the annulus deviating superiorly if the posterior half of the valvular attachment was taken as a reference point.

hearts with the usual atrial arrangement and similar morphologic features were randomly chosen. We measured the length, diameter, and location of the supporting papillary muscles within the morphologically left ventricle. The ventricular dimension measured between the apex and the crux of the heart was used to divide each value to provide standardization. The presence of a solitary papillary muscle was more frequent ($P < .01$, chi-square test) in the setting of right isomerism than in the other groups of hearts. When the papillary muscles were paired within the left ventricle, deviation of one of the papillary muscular attachments was also more frequent ($P < .05$, chi-square test) in hearts with right isomerism (Fig 6). The distance between the paired papillary muscles was significantly smaller in the group of hearts with right isomerism than in those with the usual atrial arrangement ($P < .001$, $t$-test) (Fig 7). Standardized values for the diameter and length of each papillary muscle were again significantly smaller ($P < .001$, $t$-test) in the group of hearts with right isomerism (Fig 7). These results indicate that the papillary muscles within the morphologically left ventricle are hypoplastic and dislocated in hearts with a common atrioventricular valve associated with right isomerism as compared with hearts having the usual atrial arrangement. A similar tendency was demonstrated in hearts with left isomerism, but this was not as prominent as in those with right isomerism. These structural features could be factors underscoring the insufficiency of the common atrioventricular valve and the ventricular dysfunction known to occur in patients with right isomerism. If plasty of the regurgitation valve proves to be ineffective, we suggest that it would be better to proceed directly to replacement of the valve since as yet no means exists for producing substantial papillary muscles. Moreover, preservation of the papillary muscles at the time of valvar replacement by suturing the stump of these structures to the base of the ventricle, for instance,[23, 24] is one way to produce better postoperative ventricular contractility, but care must be taken to ensure that this additional maneuver does not restrict the selection and function of available prosthetic valves.

## Circumference of the Morphologically Left Mural Leaflet

We measured the circumferential angle of the morphologically left mural leaflet in the same groups of hearts as discussed earlier. The values for the circumference were smaller in the hearts with right isomerism ($P < .001$, $t$-test) and in those with left isomerism ($P < .02$, $t$-test) than in those with the usual atrial arrangement (Fig 8). Furthermore, the circumference was significantly correlated with

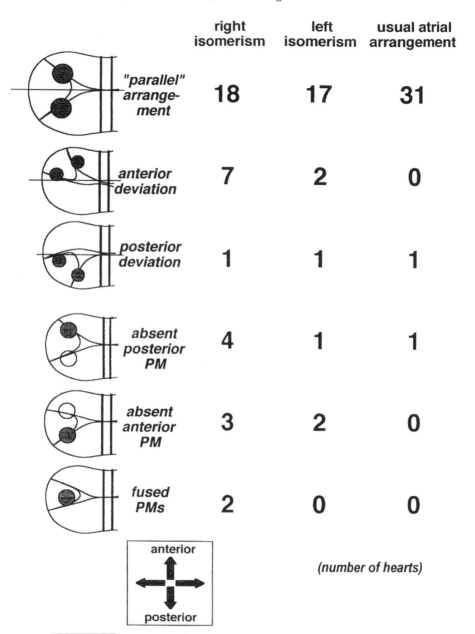

| | right isomerism | left isomerism | usual atrial arrangement |
|---|---|---|---|
| "parallel" arrangement | 18 | 17 | 31 |
| anterior deviation | 7 | 2 | 0 |
| posterior deviation | 1 | 1 | 1 |
| absent posterior PM | 4 | 1 | 1 |
| absent anterior PM | 3 | 2 | 0 |
| fused PMs | 2 | 0 | 0 |

*(number of hearts)*

**FIGURE 6.**

Arrangement of the papillary muscles. The presence of a single papillary muscle was significantly more frequent in the setting of right isomerism than in other groups of hearts. When the papillary muscles are paired within the left ventricle, deviation of one of the papillary muscular attachments was also more frequent in hearts with right isomerism.

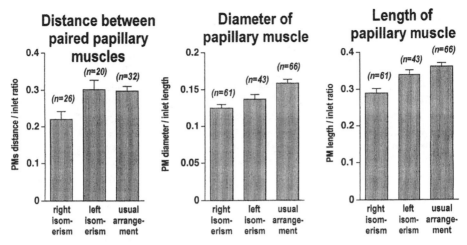

[mean value & standard erro of mean]

**FIGURE 7.**

Distances between paired papillary muscles and the diameter and length of each papillary muscle. Measured values of these features were significantly smaller in hearts with right isomerism.

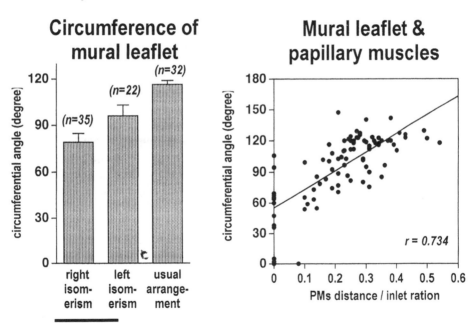

**FIGURE 8.**

Circumference of the morphologically left mural leaflet. Reflecting either the smaller distance between paired papillary muscles or the presence of a single papillary muscle, the circumferential angle of the mural leaflet within the morphologically left ventricle was significantly smaller in hearts with right isomerism.

the distance between the papillary muscular attachments, the value of the correlation coefficient being .73 (Fig 8). In the light of this finding, augmentation of the valvar leaflets by using, for example, the technique described by Kawashima and his colleagues[5] should be considered at the time of biventricular repair. Other methods for extensive valvar plasty may also be devised to supplement the size of the mural leaflet. If the mural leaflet is excessively small or even lacking, successful plasty of the morphologically left component of the atrioventricular valve combined with anatomic biventricular repair is almost impossible.

## Ventricular Proportion

Further investigations in the same series of hearts revealed that the dimension of the ventricular outlet between the apex and the attachment of the aortic valve was proportionally longer in the setting of right isomerism than in the other groups ($P < .001$, $t$-test) (Fig 9). This longer outlet-to-inlet ratio was unassociated with the presence of abnormal ventriculo-arterial connections. In contrast, the extent of septal scooping was no different among the three groups when the so-called scooped dimensions of the muscular ventricular septum were compared after standardization according to ventricular inlet length (Fig 9). These findings indicate that hearts with right isomerism have a potential for the development of obstructed aortic outflow tracts after definitive surgery. This may be enhanced by the absence of an extensively scooped muscular ventricular septum, particularly after anatomic biventricular repair involving intraventricular rerouting from the left ventricle to the aortic orifice without anterior incision of the septum. Nonetheless, when performing enlargement of a ventricular septal defect, it should be remembered that injury to the septal branch of the coronary arteries can produce severe myocardial dysfunction, as was suspected in one of our patients with left isomerism. Furthermore, not only are these situations possible during surgical maneuvers, but also the mechanism of the myocardial contraction itself might be abnormal in hearts with right isomerism because of the unusual orientation of the ventricular musculature.

## CORONARY CIRCULATION

### Coronary Arteries

As far as we know, the coronary arterial anatomy has not previously been precisely examined in hearts with isomeric appendages. In this respect, the diversity in ventricular morphology combined with abnormal ventriculo-arterial connections makes it difficult to

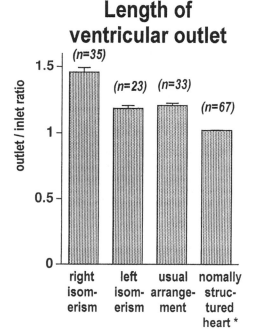

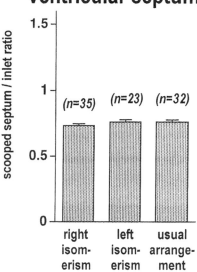

* : *Penkoske et al. (1985) [ref#34]*

**FIGURE 9.**

Ventricular shape. The ventricular outlet was proportionally longer in the setting of right isomerism than in the other groups of hearts, independent of significant differences in inlet length. The ratio in the normally structured heart was recalculated from the data demonstrated by Penkoske and her colleagues in 1986.[25]

describe simply the various patterns in coronary arterial orifices and courses. Of all of the hearts we examined, 108 with right and 54 with left isomerism were available for analysis of these anatomic features.

In 88 hearts with biventricular and ambiguous atrioventricular connections (46 with right and 42 with left isomerism), a pattern in which all major arteries arose from a solitary main stem, the so-called single coronary artery, was found in 4 (9%) and 3 (7%), respectively. The normal branching pattern, in which a short stem originating from one facing sinus gives rises to the anterior interventricular and the morphologically left circumflex arteries and the morphologically right coronary artery arises from the other facing sinus, was seen in 70% of the hearts with right isomerism and 79% of those with left isomerism. It depended on the ventricular topology and orientation of the arterial trunks as to which facing sinus gave rise to a morphologically right or left coronary artery. In the rest of the cases, a variety of patterns were seen. A common stem from one facing sinus for the anterior interventricular and the morphologically right coronary arteries and an independent origin from the other sinus for the morphologically left circumflex artery were found in 6. A similar stem for the morphologically right coronary and the left circumflex arteries was seen in 2. A pattern similar to the single coronary artery but associated with an additional branch for the right ventricle from the other facing sinus was encountered in 3, absence of the morphologically left circumflex artery in 1, a morphologically right coronary artery originating from the nonfacing sinus in 1, and dual orifices from one facing sinus in the other 3 cases, including 1 with an intramural course within the aortic wall.

A solitary coronary artery was more frequent (16%) in hearts with a dominant morphologically left ventricle and a rudimentary and incomplete morphologically right ventricle (21 with right and 4 with left isomerism). Probably related to the hypoplasia of the morphologically right ventricle, the right ventricular arteries were lacking in 9 specimens (36%). In contrast, in the reverse condition of hearts with a dominant morphologically right ventricle and a rudimentary and incomplete morphologically left ventricle (36 with right and 8 with left isomerism), the morphologically left ventricular arteries were deficient in 20 hearts (45%). The incidence of a single coronary artery in these cases was again high at 18%. Other abnormalities in the origins of the arteries from the aorta or in the proximal courses of the coronary arteries, such as an intramural course within the aortic wall and dual orifices at one sinus, were seen in 4 of 25 hearts with a dominant left ventricle and in 5 of 44 hearts with a dominant right ventricle. In the presence of a solitary and indeterminate ventricle, the nomenclature usually used for describing the major coronary arteries is inadequate for representing the arterial course. A single coronary artery was found in 3 of 6 hearts (5 with right and 1 with left isomerism). In the other 3, two major arteries originating from the facing sinuses supplied the ventricular mass in a relatively symmetrical pattern.

Although the practical implications of the high incidence of these unusual patterns remain unclear in terms of clinical features such as ventricular dysfunction, it could be helpful, in the light of potential surgical maneuvers, to know that the proximal part of the major coronary artery, or its common stems, crossed the ventricular outflow tract anterior to the arterial trunks in 26% of all the hearts we studied. Such courses would restrict any ventricular incision needed for reconstruction of an obstructed outflow tract when attempting to achieve biventricular repair.

### Cardiac Veins

In spite of the fact that the coronary sinus is universally absent in the setting of isomerism of morphologically right appendages, little attention has been directed to the venous drainage from the heart itself. Because the coronary circulation consists not only of coronary arterial perfusion but also cardiac venous drainage, the pattern and sites of venous drainage are of equal clinical importance. Our anatomic investigations on the cardiac venous system in 147 specimens, 98 with right and 49 with left isomerism, demonstrated that the system was grossly abnormal in almost all hearts with isomeric atrial appendages.

In a normal heart, the cardiac venous system consists of a circumflex part within the left atrioventricular groove and longitudinal components draining the ventricular mass. The coronary sinus, the major component of the circumflex system, commences at the origin of the oblique vein of Marshall, where it is guarded by the venous valve of Vieussens.[26-28] The left and the right coronary veins are usually located in the morphologically left and right atrioventricular grooves and are connected to the coronary sinus (Figure 10). Because of the presence of this circumflex system, all major longitudinal veins drain into the right atrial chamber via the coronary sinus, except for a few veins found on the anterior surface of the right ventricle, where a circumflex vein is usually lacking ("short cardiac veins").[26-28]

In all hearts studied with right isomerism, the coronary sinus was entirely lacking, as were the other major circumflex veins. In the group of hearts with left isomerism, the coronary sinus was present in 21 hearts (43%), including 3 in which it was unroofed. Its atrial orifice opened in the right-sided chamber in 20 and in the left-sided chamber in 1. In 6 of these hearts, one or two circumflex veins were present but were not connected to the coronary sinus. Such circumflex veins were also present in 23 hearts (47%) in which no evidence was found of the coronary sinus (see Fig 10). These independent circumflex veins had their openings adjacent to the atrioventricular junctions except for 3 cases in which an intramural course within the atrial wall produced a remote location of the orifice relative to the atrioventricular groove. The internal diameters of these circumflex veins were smaller than that of the coronary sinus. In the remaining 5 examples with left isomerism

| | circumflex component | | |
| | present | | absent |
| | coronary sinus | | |
| | present | absent | |
| isomerism of right appendages | 0 | 0 | 98 *(100%)* |
| isomerism of left appendages | 21 *(43%)* | 23 *(47%)* | 5 *(10%)* |
| presence of intramural course | 12 / 44 *(27.3%)* | | 63 / 103 *(61.2%)* |

*[number of hearts]*

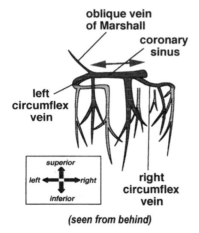

circumflex component
in normal heart

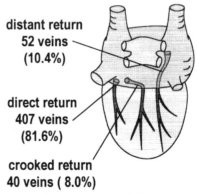

in hearts without
circumflex component

**FIGURE 10.**

Cardiac venous system. The circumflex component, including the coronary sinus defined by the presence of the oblique vein of Marshall and the venous valve of Vieussens, was entirely lacking in hearts with right isomerism. In such circumstances, longitudinal veins approaching the atria drained directly through their own orifices. Curious patterns possessing an intramural course within the atrial wall were seen in more than 60% of the hearts without any circumflex venous components.

(10%), no circumflex system could be identified, and the cardiac venous system was similar to that found in hearts with right isomerism.

In these remaining cases, all the major longitudinal veins drained directly into the atrial chambers in the absence of a circumflex system (Fig 10). This arrangement produced curious patterns of cardiac venous drainage. In these circumstances, 477 veins in 98 hearts with right isomerism and 22 in 5 with left isomerism (4.84 ± 0.95 per heart) were identified as major longitudinal veins approaching the atrial chambers from the ventricular mass. Among these, 92 veins (18.4%) followed an intramural course within the atrial wall after crossing the atrioventricular groove. Such intramural courses were seen in 63 of 103 hearts (61.2%). For 52 veins, the orifices were found within the smooth internal surface of the superior atrial component, often being adjacent to the pulmonary or hepatic venous connections to the atrium (a "distant" return) (Fig 11,A and B). In the other 40, the orifices were in the spaces between the pectinate muscles, the intramural course running along the atrioventricular groove (a "crooked" return). Intramural or crooked terminations were found more frequently in the posterior aspect of the cardiac mass (51% of the abnormal courses) than in the anterior (27%) or lateral (22%) parts. The other longitudinal veins without an intramural course drained directly into the atrial chamber through the space between the pectinate muscles near the atrioventricular junction (a "direct" return).

In the group of 44 hearts with left isomerism and a circumflex venous system, drainage from their longitudinal veins was frequently into the circumflex veins or the coronary sinus (180 of all of the 260 longitudinal veins identified, 69%). Still, however, 66 longitudinal veins (25%) had their own orifices producing a direct connection, and 14 veins (seen in 12 hearts, 27% of this group) followed an intramural course before draining into the atrial chambers.

In terms of the surgical implications of these abnormalities in the cardiac venous system, attention should first be paid to the intramural course. An abnormal course may be damaged by the surgeon either at the time of the initial atriotomy or when making extensive atrial incisions for maneuvers such as intra-atrial rerouting or repair of totally anomalous pulmonary venous connections. Indeed, we identified such direct surgical damage on distant venous return during our investigation, although it is not clear whether the injuries were of major importance in the death of the patients. Abnormal courses are also of significance with regard to postopera-

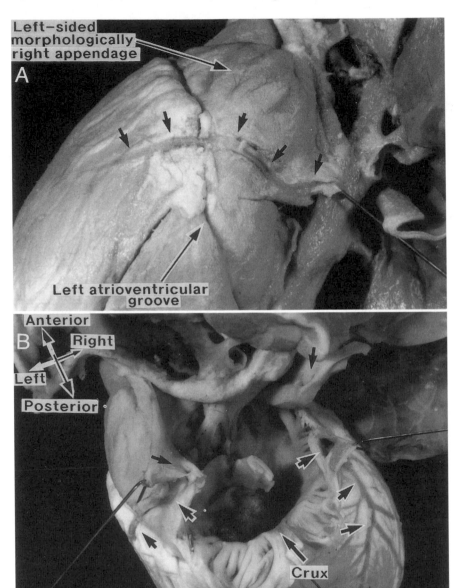

**FIGURE 11.**

**A,** distant return of a longitudinal cardiac vein *(arrows)*. As far as our investigations are concerned, we have never encountered this sort of intramural course of cardiac veins in either normal hearts or malformed hearts with the usual atrial arrangement. **B,** intramural courses and orifices for

*(Continued.)*

tive occlusion of the cardiac venous orifices by an intra-atrial thrombus. The openings through the spaces between the pectinate muscles seem to be readily obstructed. Postoperative anticoagulation therapy will therefore play an important role in avoiding unfavorable thrombosis. In addition, we speculate that different cardiac venous pressures within the heart after a Fontan-type operation might be of functional significance. Some of the individual drainages of the longitudinal veins can be directed to the high-pressure pathway and others to the low-pressure atrial chamber. In these circumstances, the myocardial perfusion would, theoretically speaking, be unbalanced. Because of this, our preference is to construct a total cavopulmonary connection, thus placing all the venous drainage into the low-pressure chamber.

All these considerations would nonetheless likely produce no significant difference in patients with stable postoperative hemodynamics because alternative venous drainage via collateral pathways will probably be formed more quickly than for the arterial supply. In the acute phase after invasive surgical procedures, however, functionally or anatomically obstructed drainage of the cardiac veins could have unwanted deleterious effects on ventricular function, particularly myocardial edema.

## IMPLICATIONS FOR THE SINUS NODE AND THE CONDUCTION SYSTEM

Extensive intra-atrial maneuvers are likely to have a greater probability of injuring the sinus node than simple surgical options. In the setting of right isomerism, it is well established that the sinus node is duplicated, being located bilaterally at the junctions between the superior caval veins and the atria.[3, 29, 30] In contrast, the sinus node is histologically hypoplastic or even absent in hearts with left isomerism.[30] An inferior location for the earliest site of atrial activation is the most common pattern in this setting.[31, 32] In our clinical experience of epicardial mapping during surgery in 23 patients with left isomerism, the earliest site of activation was most

---

**FIGURE 11 (cont.).**

distant returns. Such terminations of the cardiac veins were found more frequently in the posterior aspect of the cardiac mass than in the anterior or lateral parts. The orifices *(large arrows)* were found within the smooth internal surface of the superior atrial wall, often being adjacent to the pulmonary or hepatic venous connections to the atrium. Note the presence of trabeculations on the posterior atrial walls.

frequently identified at the junction between a hepatic vein and the atrium (57%).[33] These sites of earliest activation can be injured not only by extensive intra-atrial procedures but also by inattentive cannulation into the hepatic vein when establishing cardiopulmonary bypass. Our preference when establishing a total cavopulmonary connection is to place either the sinus node or the site of earliest activation into the low-pressure instead of the high-pressure pathway.[9] This is because a pacemaker placed within the high-pressure chamber might produce chronotropic abnormalities in the long term and affect the response to exercise or enhance the occurrence of atrial arrhythmia. With all these problems in mind, it is crucial to have knowledge regarding both the precise location of the sinus node and the earliest site of atrial activation.

The location of the atrioventricular node is also of surgical importance. As has been described, surgical treatment on regurgitant atrioventricular valves can be crucial in both the short and long term after definitive surgery. The efficacy of annuloplasty would likely be mitigated if a surgical atrioventricular block developed. Although the number of articles describing morphologic findings is still small,[29, 30] it is known that a posterior node is the rule in hearts with a right-hand ventricular topology whereas an anterior node or a sling is expected in hearts with left-hand topology, both of these locations being related to the junction with the crest of the muscular ventricular septum. In hearts with a dominant right ventricle and an incomplete left ventricle, the atrioventricular node usually gives rise to a conducting bundle at the posterior crest of the muscular ventricular septum. In all other circumstances, the node is related to an anterior course of the penetrating bundle. When the ventricular mass is formed by a solitary and indeterminate chamber, the location of the conduction tissue cannot be reliably predicted.

## SUMMARY

As we have tried to demonstrate in this chapter, extensive understanding of morphology is necessary for successful definitive repair in individual patients with isomeric atrial appendages, as well as for the further evolution of optimal surgical strategies. Obviously different from patients with the usual atrial arrangement, those with isomeric atrial appendages have specific morphologic features that may underscore the clinical problems frequently found in this setting. Surgical strategies as well as individual operative procedures should be established on the basis of knowledge regarding those features presently demonstrated, namely, ventricular structures, the atrioventricular valves, the coronary circulation, and so on. Further investigations will certainly provide other aspects of which we are at present unaware.

### ACKNOWLEDGMENT

This work could not have been performed without the help and support of many friends and colleagues. In particular, we express our gratitude to Siew Yen Ho, Audrey Smith, and William A. Devine.

## REFERENCES

1. Abernethy J: Account of two instances of uncommon formations in the viscera of the human body. *Philosoph Trans* 83:59–66, 1793.
2. Martin MG: Observation d'une deviation organique de l'estomac d'une anomalie dans la situation dans la configuration du coeur et des vaisseaux qui en partent ou qui s'y rendant. *Bull Soc Anat Paris* 1:39–43, 1826.
3. Van Mierop LHS, Wiglesworth FW: Isomerism of the cardiac atria in the asplenia syndrome. *Lab Invest* 11:1303–1315, 1962.
4. Moller JH, Nakib A, Anderson RC, et al: Congenital cardiac disease associated with polysplenia: A developmental complex of bilateral "left-sideness." *Circulation* 36:789–799, 1967.
5. Kawashima Y, Matsuda H, Naito Y, et al: Biventricular repair of cardiac isomerism with common atrioventricular canal with the aid of an endocardial cushion prosthesis. *J Thorac Cardiovasc Surg* 106:248–254, 1993.
6. Pacifico AD, Ricchi A, Bargeron LMJ, et al: Corrective repair of complete atrioventricular canal defects and major associated cardiac anomalies. *Ann Thorac Surg* 46:645–651, 1988.
7. Ando F, Shirotani H, Kawai J, et al: Successful total repair of complicated cardiac anomalies with asplenia syndrome. *J Thorac Cardiovasc Surg* 72:33–38, 1976.
8. Humes RA, Feldt RH, Porter CJ, et al: The modified Fontan operation for asplenia and polysplenia syndrome. *J Thorac Cardiovasc Surg* 96:212–218, 1988.
9. Yagihara T, Kishimoto H, Isobe F, et al: Indication and result of right heart bypass operation (in Japanese). *Jpn J Cardiovasc Surg* 20:1389–1392, 1991.
10. Driscoll DJ, Offord KP, Felt RH, et al: Five- to fifteen-year follow-up after Fontan operation. *Circulation* 85:469–496, 1992.
11. Uemura H, Yagihara T, Kawashima Y, et al: What affects ventricular characteristics after a Fontan type operation (abstract)? Presented at the 74th Annual Meeting of the American Association for Thoracic Surgery, 1994, New York, 1994, p 170.

12. Kawashima Y, Kitamura S, Matsuda H, et al: Total cavopulmonary shunt operation in complex cardiac anomalies: A new operation. *J Thorac Cardiovasc Surg* 87:74–81, 1984.

13. Hopkins RA, Armstrong BE, Serwer GA, et al: Physiological rationale for a bidirectional cavopulmonary shunt: A versatile complement to the Fontan principle. *J Thorac Cardiovasc Surg* 90:391–398, 1985.

14. Mazzera E, Corno A, Picardo S, et al: Bidirectional cavopulmonary shunts: Clinical applications as staged or definitive palliation. *Ann Thorac Surg* 47:415–420, 1989.

15. Bridges ND, Jonas RA, Mayer JE, et al: Bidirectional cavopulmonary anastomosis as interim palliation for high-risk Fontan candidates: Early results. *Circulation* 82(suppl 4):170–176, 1990.

16. Douville EC, Sade RM, Fyfe DA: Hemi-Fontan operation in surgery for single ventricle: A preliminary report. *Ann Thorac Surg* 51:893–900, 1991.

17. Van Praagh R, Van Praagh S: Atrial isomerism in the heterotaxy syndromes with asplenia, or polysplenia, or normally formed spleen: An erroneous concept. *Am J Cardiol* 66:1504–1506, 1990.

18. Phoon CK, Neil CA: Asplenia syndrome: Insight into embryology through an analysis of cardiac and extracardiac anomalies. *Am J Cardiol* 73:581–587, 1994.

19. Kirklin JW, Barratt-Boyes BG: Atrial isomerism, in Kirklin JW, Barratt-Boyes BG (eds): *Cardiac Surgery*, vol 2, ed 2. New York, Churchill Livingstone, 1993, pp 1585–1596.

20. Le Feuvre C, Metzger JP, Lachurie ML, et al: Treatment of severe mitral regurgitation caused by ischemic papillary muscle dysfunction: Indications for coronary angioplasty. *Am Heart J* 123:860–865, 1992.

21. Sarris GE, Miller DC: Valvular-ventricular interaction: The importance of the mitral chordae tendineae in terms of global left ventricular systolic function. *J Card Surg* 3:215–234, 1988.

22. Yun KL, Fann JI, Rayhill SC, et al: Importance of the mitral subvalvular apparatus for left ventricular segmental systolic mechanics. *Circulation* 82(suppl 4):89–104, 1990.

23. Miki S, Kusuhara K, Ueda Y, et al: Mitral valve replacement with preservation of chordae tendineae and papillary muscles. *Ann Thorac Surg* 45:28–34, 1988.

24. David TE, Burns RJ, Bacchus CM, et al: Mitral valve replacement for mitral regurgitation with and without preservation of chordae tendineae. *J Thorac Cardiovasc Surg* 88:718–725, 1984.

25. Penkoske PA, Neches WH, Anderson RH, et al: Further observations on the morphology of atrioventricular septal defects. *J Thorac Cardiovasc Surg* 90:611–622, 1985.

26. Walmsley T: Blood vessels of the heart, in Sharpey-Schafer E, Symington J, Bryce TH (eds): *Quain's Elements of Anatomy*, vol 4, ed 11. *The Heart*. London, Longmans Green, 1929, pp 98–109.

27. Gross L: The veins of the heart, in Gross L (ed): *The Blood Supply to the Heart.* New York, Paul B Hoeber, 1921, pp 93–104.

28. Mochizuki S: Vv. cordis (in German), in Adachi B (ed): *Anatomie der Japaner II, Das Venensystem der Japaner, erste Lieferung.* Tokyo, Verlag der Kaiserlich-Japanischen Universitaet zu Kyoto, Kenkyusha, 1933, pp 41–64.

29. Ho SY, Fagg N, Anderson RH, et al: Disposition of the atrioventricular conduction tissues in the heart with isomerism of the atrial appendages. Its relation to congenital complete heart block. *J Am Coll Cardiol* 20:904–910, 1991.

30. Dickinson DF, Wilkinson JL, Anderson KR, et al: The cardiac conduction system in situs ambiguous. *Circulation* 59:879–885, 1979.

31. Momma K, Takao A, Shibata T: Characteristics and natural history of abnormal atrial rhythms in left isomerism. *Am J Cardiol* 65:231–236, 1990.

32. Wren C, Macartney FJ, Deanfield JE: Cardiac rhythm in atrial isomerism. *Am J Cardiol* 59:1156–1158, 1987.

33. Uemura H, Yagihara T, Yamamoto F, et al: Where is sinus node in hearts with isomeric appendages (abstract)? *J Am Coll Cardiol* p 192A, 1994.

# Management of the Anomalous Origin of the Left Coronary Artery From the Pulmonary Artery

**Abbas Ardehali, M.D.**
Division of Cardiothoracic Surgery, Department of Surgery, UCLA Medical Center, Los Angeles, California

**Hillel Laks, M.D.**
Division of Cardiothoracic Surgery, Department of Surgery, UCLA Medical Center, Los Angeles, California

**Vivekanand Allada, M.D.**
Division of Pediatric Cardiology, Department of Pediatrics, UCLA Medical Center, Los Angeles, California

---

A nomalous origin of the left coronary artery from the pulmonary artery (ALCA) is a rare congenital anomaly; the incidence is estimated to be 1 in every 300,000 live births.[1] In children with congenital heart disease undergoing cardiac catheterization, ALCA is identified in 1 of 400 patients.[2] Morphologically, ALCA arises most commonly from the sinus above the left or posterior cusp of the pulmonary valve. Less frequently, ALCA is connected to the right aspect of the pulmonary artery. In utero and early in postnatal life, this congenital anomaly may remain undiagnosed because the pulmonary artery pressure is high enough to perfuse the anomalous coronary artery. Clinical manifestation of this lesion depends on its anatomic and hemodynamic variables. As pulmonary artery pressure falls in early postnatal life, myocardial perfusion via the ALCA decreases. This decrease in coronary perfusion pressure can result in myocardial ischemia. Furthermore, development of significant collaterals can shunt blood from the right coronary artery to the low-pressure pulmonary artery via the ALCA. This may result in congestive heart failure from the left-to-right shunt and/or myocardial ischemia from the coronary steal phenomenon.

The clinical syndrome of ALCA was first described by Bland,

White, and Garland in 1933, and it continues to bear their names.[3] The clinical characteristics of infants with an anomalous left coronary artery may include poor feeding, breathlessness and sweating upon feeding, growth retardation, and congestive heart failure. Symptoms in early infancy (younger than 2 months) are rare as a result of high postnatal pulmonary artery pressure minimizing the runoff into the pulmonary artery. On examination, infants with ALCA frequently have electrocardiographic evidence of myocardial infarction and left ventricular (LV) hypertrophy. They may have severe mitral regurgitation and may be in cardiogenic shock (because of the absence of adequate collateral circulation). Patients with ALCA who are seen in adulthood have had significant right coronary artery collateral circulation to the left coronary artery territory to minimize myocardial ischemia; their symptoms in later stages of life may include fatigue, exertional angina, myocardial infarction, and congestive heart failure.

## PREOPERATIVE DIAGNOSTIC STUDIES

The definitive diagnosis of ALCA has conventionally required cardiac catheterization and coronary angiography. An aortogram may demonstrate a single right coronary artery arising from the aortic root, with runoff of contrast into the left coronary artery through the collateral circulation and opacification of the main pulmonary artery. A left ventriculogram provides an assessment of residual ventricular function and demonstrates the degree of mitral regurgitation. Depending on the degree of shunting, there may be a step-up in arterial oxygen saturation in the main pulmonary artery.

Echocardiography is a useful diagnostic modality in patients with ALCA. Two-dimensional and pulsed Doppler echocardiography with color flow mapping can demonstrate continuity of the left coronary artery with the pulmonary trunk and detect retrograde flow through the coronary artery into the pulmonary artery. A recent prospective study yielded no false-positive or false-negative diagnoses in patients with ALCA, in expert hands.[4] These infants underwent surgical repair based only on the echocardiographic diagnoses. Karr et al. have also demonstrated that two echocardiographic findings can be reliably used for the diagnosis of ALCA: (1) detection of an abnormal jet into the pulmonary trunk and (2) retrograde flow in at least one segment of the left coronary artery system.[5] The role of transesophageal echocardiography in the diagnosis of ALCA remains to be established. It has been reported that transesophageal echocardiography can provide clear anatomic information in infants with ALCA when transthoracic echocardiography is inconclusive.[6]

Although the gold standard for the diagnosis of ALCA remains cardiac catheterization and cinecardiography, experience with two-dimensional and Doppler echocardiography with color flow mapping is accumulating. At the present time, surgical intervention can be undertaken based on echocardiographic findings in selected cases.

## SURGICAL TREATMENT

The diagnosis of ALCA in an infant, usually critically ill, or an adult is an indication for urgent surgical treatment. Surgical treatment of ALCA has undergone significant evolution in the past 40 years. Procedures such as creation of an aortopulmonary fistula to increase saturation of the pulmonary artery, banding of the pulmonary artery, and pericardial poudrage are only of historical interest.[7–9] The ideal operation, in nearly all patients, is construction of a two–coronary artery system. The methods for creation of a two–coronary artery system include reimplantation of the ALCA, an aortopulmonary tunnel operation (Takeuchi repair), subclavian-to–left coronary artery anastomosis, and coronary artery bypass grafting (using an internal mammary or vein graft).

Irrespective of the type of operation planned, it is of utmost importance that proper preoperative and intraoperative measures be undertaken for optimal myocardial preservation. Because of pre-existing myocardial ischemia, ventricular fibrillation may occur before cannulation and cardiopulmonary bypass. Thus preoperatively, the hemodynamic state should be optimized and cannulation should be performed without touching the ventricles, if at all possible, because of vulnerability of the myocardium to ventricular fibrillation.

During the administration of cardioplegic solution, the pulmonary artery trunk or the origin of the left coronary artery should be occluded to prevent runoff of the solution into the low-pressure pulmonary artery system and ensure uniform delivery to the myocardium. We routinely use cold intermittent antegrade/retrograde cardioplegia with a terminal warm dose. Left ventricular assist devices have been and should be used perioperatively when systemic perfusion is compromised because of the reversible nature of myocardial ischemic dysfunction and the high likelihood of functional recovery.[10, 11]

Reimplantation of the ALCA into the lateral wall of the aorta is considered the operation of choice, if technically feasible.[12] For reimplantation of the ALCA, a generous vertical incision on the pulmonary artery trunk is made to allow direct visualization of the origin of the left coronary artery (Fig 1, A). The ALCA is excised with a button of pulmonary artery and mobilized for a short distance to allow a tension-free anastomosis to the left lateral wall of the aorta (Fig 1, B). Next, an anterior aortotomy is made and a button of aorta from the left sinus removed. The anterior aortotomy

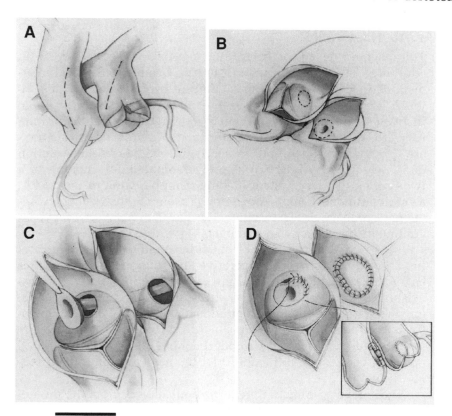

**FIGURE 1.**

The technique of aortic implantation of anomalous left coronary artery. **A,** an incision is made on the pulmonary artery trunk to visualize the origin of the left coronary artery. A vertical incision is also made on ascending aorta. **B,** The ALCA is excised with a button of pulmonary artery trunk. **C,** the ALCA is mobilized and is passed through a button of aorta that has been removed from the left sinus. **D,** the anastomosis is performed under direct visualization from inside the aorta; the opening in the pulmonary artery is closed with a pericardial patch. (From Laks H, Ardehali A, Grant PW, et al: *J Thorac Cardiovasc Surg* 109:519–523, 1995. Used by permission.)

provides optimal exposure and allows optimal reimplantation of the ALCA just above the left sinus, without potential injury to the valvular apparatus (Fig 1, C). The ALCA with a button of pulmonary artery is pulled into the aorta and sutured in place from inside (Fig 1, D). The sinus of the pulmonary artery is reconstructed with a pericardial patch, and the vertical openings in the aorta and pulmonary artery are repaired primarily.

Several techniques for prolongation of the anomalous coronary artery to allow a tension-free anastomosis to the aorta have been described. These include tube extension of the left coronary artery with excised pulmonary artery tissue or a combination of the cuff of the pulmonary artery and an excised aortic flap.[13, 14] Long-term follow-up of patients who have undergone these coronary prolongation techniques is not yet available.

Direct reimplantation of the ALCA is not technically possible in all patients. In cases where the ALCA origin is too distant from the ascending aorta and coronary prolongation techniques are deemed unsafe, aortocoronary continuity can be established within the lumen of the pulmonary artery with a baffle constructed from the native pulmonary artery tissue (Takeuchi repair).[15] In this procedure, an aortopulmonary window is created and sutured. An anterior pulmonary artery flap is created, and the tunnel inside the pulmonary artery is constructed between the aortopulmonary window and the left coronary artery ostium by suturing the pulmonary arterial flap to the posterior wall of the pulmonary artery trunk. The anterior pulmonary artery flap may be medially or laterally based, depending on technical ease. The pulmonary artery anterior wall defect is then reconstructed with a pericardial patch. The Takeuchi technique has proved to be a simple, yet effective method of establishing aortocoronary continuity.

The other two methods for creation of a two–coronary artery system are a subclavian-to–left coronary artery anastomosis and coronary artery bypass grafting. The advantage of an end-to-end subclavian–left coronary artery anastomosis is that it can be performed without cardiopulmonary bypass in critically ill patients with poor ventricular function.[16] However, potential problems with use of the subclavian artery are kinking of the artery at its origin, upper extremity ischemia, and anastomotic stenosis. Backer et al. identified severe anastomotic stenosis in two of five patients who underwent subclavian-to–coronary artery anastomosis in late follow-up; reoperation was required for coronary revascularization.[17] The use of saphenous vein grafts for coronary artery bypass in infants is limited because of the small caliber of the grafts. The internal mammary artery has also been anastomosed to the left coronary artery with good short-term patency.[18] In critically ill infants with a substantial left-to-right shunt, simple ligation of the ALCA can occasionally be justified. In such cases, follow-up clinical or laboratory documentation of myocardial ischemia should lead to revascularization of the left coronary artery.

## CONCOMITANT SURGICAL PROCEDURES

Patients with ALCA may have moderate to severe mitral regurgitation and/or an LV aneurysm. Mitral insufficiency is related to both anatomic distortion of the valvular apparatus as a result of LV dilation as well as ischemic damage to the papillary muscles. The need for simultaneous surgical treatment of these entities remains controversial. It is reassuring to note that damaged infant myocardium has great regenerating potential. Re-establishment of oxygenated coronary blood flow to the LV myocardium has been shown to substantially improve LV function and shape.[19] In infants, significant grades of mitral regurgitation have been shown to regress spontaneously, and dyskinetic segments of myocardium have regained function.[20] Thus it appears prudent that in infants, only severe mitral regurgitation should be surgically treated simultaneously. In adults, we have a lower threshold for repairing mitral valve insufficiency. Resection of LV dyskinetic segments is a very rare occurrence in our experience.

## RISK FACTORS FOR PERIOPERATIVE MORTALITY

Perioperative mortality in patients with ALCA ranges from 0% to 75%, primarily because of population heterogeneity and small sample sizes of the reported series. In 1981, Laborde et al. analyzed their experience in patients with ALCA and found a high operative mortality in younger adults.[21] As experience with surgical treatment accumulated, it became evident that delaying coronary revascularization is hazardous because of progressive myocardial injury and sudden death. Multiple subsequent reports have concluded that young age is no longer a contraindication for surgical intervention and revascularization should be undertaken urgently upon diagnosis.[22-24]

The severity of preoperative LV dysfunction appears to be the most important risk factor for mortality. Sauer et al. analyzed the risk factors for perioperative mortality in 33 children with ALCA over a period of 18 years.[25] The extent of myocardial ischemia as well as young age proved to be the two important risk factors for mortality at corrective surgery. As noted earlier, coronary revascularization is no longer delayed because of the age of an infant. Vouhe et al. observed a 31% mortality rate in patients with an LV shortening fraction of less than 0.20 vs. 0% mortality among patients with an LV shortening fraction of 0.20 or more (P = 0.03).[22] Thus preoperative LV function is highly predictive of perioperative mortality. Optimization of the hemodynamic state preoperatively, improvement in intraoperative myocardial preservation techniques, and judicious use of refined LV assist devices can further enhance the results of surgical treatment in this group of patients.

## LONG-TERM FOLLOW-UP
### CONTRACTILE FUNCTION
Despite the severity of preoperative systolic dysfunction, LV function in both infants and older patients with ALCA is significantly improved after corrective surgery. There is a reduction in the cardiothoracic ratio,[26] an increase in the LV shortening fraction and ejection fraction,[19] and a reduction in LV end-diastolic and systolic volume.[27] Further evaluation with nuclear single proton emission computed tomography perfusion imaging has demonstrated restoration of coronary blood flow after surgery.[28]

### CONDUIT PATENCY/PROCEDURAL COMPLICATIONS
Conduit patency is an important end point that has been incompletely studied in most long-term follow-up reports. Patency can not be assumed because of the patient's lack of symptoms since there are many patients with a one–coronary artery system who are asymptomatic. Follow-up studies of the direct reimplantation technique have been encouraging. Vouhe et al. followed 23 perioperative survivors of direct aortic reimplantation for 4.4 ± 2.5 years and found patency of the reimplanted anomalous left coronary artery in each patient.[22] Neirotti et al. also found that the reimplanted left coronary artery was patent in each of the reevaluated patients (10 of 12 patients).[29] Other series have also confirmed the long-term patency of reimplanted coronary arteries with minimal late morbidity or need for reoperations.[19, 30]

The late complications of aortopulmonary window creation with an intrapulmonary baffle include supravalvular pulmonary stenosis, an obstructed aortocoronary tunnel, and a residual baffle leak into the pulmonary artery. Bunton et al. reviewed their experience with 11 patients who underwent the Takeuchi procedure over a mean follow-up period of 18½ months.[31] They observed two cases of supravalvular pulmonary stenosis (one requiring a second operation), one case of an asymptomatic obstructed baffle, and the development of mild aortic regurgitation in one patient. There were no early or late deaths in the group of patients who underwent the Takeuchi procedure. Thrombosis of the intrapulmonary baffle was also reported in one of four patients who underwent this procedure by Tkebuchava et al.[32] Because of the potential late complications, we employ the Takeuchi procedure as an alternate method of establishing a two–coronary artery system in patients in whom direct reimplantation of the ALCA is not technically possible.

In summary, ALCA is a rare congenital heart lesion that should be surgically treated once a diagnosis is made. Advances in echocardiographic techniques and instrumentation may allow a definitive diagnosis of ALCA noninvasively in the near future. The goals of surgical management are establishment of a two–coronary artery system with long-term patency and using native tissue to allow for normal growth of the anastomosis. Accumulating data suggest the long-term superiority of reimplantation of the ALCA to other methods for re-establishment of a two–coronary artery system. When reimplantation of the left coronary artery is not technically possible, the Takeuchi procedure has been shown to be a simple and effective method of establishing a two–coronary artery system. The severity of myocardial dysfunction is the most important risk factor for perioperative mortality. Advances in perioperative care and myocardial preservation techniques and the availability of LV assist devices may further improve the results of surgical treatment of ALCA.

## REFERENCES

1. Keith JD: The anomalous origin of the left coronary artery from the pulmonary artery. *Br Heart J* 21:149–161, 1959.
2. Askenazi J, Nadas AS: Anomalous left coronary artery originating from the pulmonary artery. Report on 15 cases. Circulation 51:976–987, 1975.
3. Bland EF, White PD, Garland J: Congenital anamolies of the coronary arteries: Report of an unsual case associated with cardiac hypertrophy. *Am Heart J* 8:787–801, 1933.
4. Jureidini SB, Nouri S, Crawford CJ, et al: Reliability of echocardiography in the diagnosis of anomalous origin of the left coronary artery from the pulmonary trunk. *Am Heart J* 122:61–88, 1991.
5. Karr SS, Parness IA, Sperak PJ, et al: Diagnosis of anomalous left coronary artery by Doppler color flow mapping: Distinction from other

causes of dilated cardiomyopathy. *J Am Coll Cardiol* 17:1271–1275, 1992.

6. Kececioglu D, Kotthoff S, Konertz W, et al: Pulmonary artery origin of the left coronary artery: Diagnosis by transesophageal echocardiography in infancy. *Eru Heart J* 14:1006–1007, 1993.

7. Gasul BM, Loeflfleer ME: Anomalous origin of the left coronary artery from the pulmonary artery (Bland-Garland-White syndrome): Report of 4 cases. *Pediatrics* 4:498–501, 1949.

8. Case RB, Morrow AG, Stainsby W, et al: Anomalous origin of the left coronary artery. *Circulation* 17:1062–1068, 1958.

9. Paul RN, Robbins SG: A surgical treatment proposed for either endocardial fibroelastosis or anomalous left coronary artery. *Pediatrics* 47:196, 1955.

10. Taub JO, Klinedienst WJ, Pennington DG: Case report: Left ventricular assistance in a two month old following repair of an anomalous left coronary artery. *Proc Acad Cardiopulmon Perfusion* 9:162–164, 1988.

11. Dua R, Smith JA, Wilkinson JL, et al: Long term follow-up after two coronary repair of anomalous left coronary artery from the pulmonary artery. *J Cardiac Surg* 8:384–390, 1993.

12. Laks H, Ardehali A, Grant PW et al: Aortic reimplantation of anomalous left coronary artery: An improved surgical approach. *J Thorac Cardiovasc Surg* 109:716–720, 1995.

13. Sese A, Imoto Y: New technique in the transfer of an anomalously originated left coronary artery to the aorta. *Ann Thorac Surg* 53:527–529, 1992.

14. Vingeswaran WT, Campbell DN, Pappas G, et al: Evolution of the management of anomalous left coronary artery: A new surgical approach. *Ann Thorac Surg* 48:560–564, 1989.

15. Takeuchi S, Imamura H, Katsumoto K, et al: New surgical method for repair of anomalous left coronary artery from pulmonary artery. *J Thorac Cardiovasc Surg* 78:7–11, 1979.

16. Meyer BW, Stefanik G, Stiles QR, et al: A method of definitive surgical treatment of anomalous origin of left coronary artery. *J Thorac Cardiovasc Surg* 56:104–107, 1968.

17. Backer CL, Stout MJ, Zales VR, et al: Anomalous origin of the left coronary artery: Twenty years review of surgical management. *J Thorac Cardiovasc Surg* 103:1049–1058, 1992.

18. Kitamura S, Kawachi K, Nishii T, et al: Internal thoracic artery grafting for congenital coronary malformations. *Ann Thorac Surg* 53:513–516, 1992.

19. Carvalho JS, Redington AN, Oldershaw PJ, et al: Analysis of left ventricular wall movement before and after reimplantation of anomalous left coronary artery in infancy. *Br Heart J* 65:218–222, 1991.

20. Menahem S, Venables AW: Anomalous left coronary artery from the pulmonary artery: A 15 year sample. *Br Heart J* 58:378–384, 1987.

21. Laborde F, Marchand M, Leca F, et al: Surgical treatment of anoma-

lous origin of the left coronary artery in infancy and childhood. Early and late results in 20 consecutive cases. *J Thorac Cardiovasc Surg* 82:423–428, 1981.

22. Vouhe PR, Tamisier D, Sidi D, et al: Anomalous left coronary artery from the pulmonary artery: Results of isolated aortic reimplantation. *Ann Thorac Surg* 54:621–626, 1992.

23. Guikahue MK, Sidi D, Kachaner J, et al: Anomalous left coronary artery arising from the pulmonary artery in infancy: Is early operation better? *Br Heart J* 60:522–526, 1988.

24. Wollenek G, Domanig E, Salzer-Muhar U, et al: Anomalous origin of the left coronary artery: A review of surgical management in 13 patients. *J Cardiovasc Surg* 34:399–405, 1993.

25. Sauer U, Stern H, Meisner H, et al: Risk factors for perioperative mortality in children with anomalous origin of the left coronary artery from the pulmonary artery. *J Thorac Cardiovasc Surg* 104:696–705, 1992.

26. Arciniegas E, Farooki ZQ, Hakimi M, et al: Management of anomalous left coronary artery from the pulmonary artery. *Circulation* 62(suppl 1):180–189, 1980.

27. Jin Z, Berger F, Uhlemann F, et al: Improvement in left ventricular dysfunction after aortic reimplantation in 11 consecutive paediatric patients with anomalous origin of the left coronary artery from the pulmonary artery. Early results of a serial echocardiographic follow-up. *Eur Heart J* 15:1044–1049, 1994.

28. Stern H, Sauer U, Locher D, et al: Left ventricular function assessed with echocardiography and myocardial perfusion assessed with scintigraphy under dipyridamole stress in pediatric patients after repair for anomalous origin of the left coronary artery from the pulmonary artery. *J Thorac Cardiovasc Surg* 106:723–732, 1993.

29. Neirotti R, Nijveld A, Ithuralde M, et al: Anomalous origin of the left coronary artery from the pulmonary artery: Repair by aortic reimplantation. *Eur J Cardiothorac Surg* 5:368–371, 1991.

30. Alexi-Meskisvili V, Hetzer R, Weng Y, et al: Anomalous origin of the left coronary artery from the pulmonary artery. Early results with direct aortic reimplantation. *J Thorac Cardiovasc Surg* 108:354–362, 1994.

31. Bunton R, Jonas RA, Lang P, et al: Anomalous origin of the left coronary artery from the pulmonary artery: Ligation versus establishment of a two coronary artery system. *J Thorac Cardiovasc Surg* 93:103–108, 1987.

32. Tkebuchava T, Carrel T, von Sagesser L, et al: Repair of anomalous origin of the left coronary artery from the pulmonary artery without early and late mortality in 9 patients. *J Cardiovasc Surg* 33:479–485, 1992.

# Approaches to Sternal Wound Infections

**Lawrence J. Gottlieb, M.D.**
Professor of Clinical Surgery, Section of Plastic and Reconstructive Surgery, University of Chicago, Chicago, Illinois

**Elisabeth K. Beahm, M.D.**
Chief Resident, Section of Plastic and Reconstructive Surgery, University of Chicago, Chicago, Illinois

**Thomas J. Krizek, M.D.**
Professor of Surgery, Vice-Chairman of the Department of Surgery and Chief of Plastic Surgery, University of South Florida, Tampa, Florida

**Robert B. Karp, M.D.**
Professor of Surgery, Chief of Cardiac Surgery, University of Chicago, Pritzker School of Medicine, Chicago, Illinois

A median sternotomy provides an approach to the heart and great vessels with unparalleled access and minimal interference with respiration. Sternotomy wounds are large wounds, often associated with long operations, and are complicated by considerable blood loss or hematoma. The incision divides the superficially located sternum, a bone subject to the constant motion and stress of breathing. The sternum is difficult to immobilize even with large amounts of foreign body (wire). It should therefore not be surprising that some sternal wounds become infected and demonstrate bony dehiscence.

Mediastinitis occurs in 1% to 2.5% of patients who undergo median sternotomy, the prevalence unchanged for more than 20 years.[1-12] It is a life-threatening condition. Valvular procedures carry a rate of infection of 1.8%, slightly higher than coronary artery bypass procedures. When these two procedures are done concomitantly, the rate of mediastinitis is 2.5% to 3%.[3] Use of a single internal mammary artery (IMA) may increase the incidence of infection, and when both arteries are used, the infection rate approaches 5%.[13] In contrast, the reported incidence of suppurative mediastinitis in children undergoing cardiac procedures is less than 1%.[14] The mortality of suppurative mediastinitis is reported to be nearly 100% without treatment.

*Advances in Cardiac Surgery®*, vol. 7
© 1996, Mosby–Year Book, Inc.

Refinements in the operative management of sternal wound infection have drastically reduced mortality rates. We will review the principles that guide our treatment of mediastinitis as well as our experience with sternal salvage based on clinical assessment of sternal vascularity, osseous quantitative bacteriology, and rigid fixation in patients with post–median sternotomy mediastinitis.

# PATHOGENESIS OF INFECTION

Surgical infections do not result from the mere presence of bacteria, but rather from a complex interplay between the host's (patient) available systemic and local defense mechanisms and pathogenic microorganisms. Experience in burns and other contaminated wounds indicates that a bacterial count of $10^5$ microorganisms per gram of tissue is a critical level. Counts less than this allow successful wound closure.[15] Higher levels cause breakdown and, as bacterial counts increase, may lead to invasive sepsis. It is important to examine those factors in both the patient and the operation that might allow levels to reach $10^5$ microorganisms per gram.

## PREDISPOSING PATIENT FACTORS

A review of the literature reveals a seemingly endless list of risk factors for the development of post–median sternotomy mediastinitis. These factors may be categorized as preoperative, intraoperative, and postoperative risk factors.

### Preoperative Risk Factors

Logically, patients who are initially ill, as manifested by a poor nutritional or hemodynamic status or who are undergoing reoperation, have adverse factors that predispose to infection. Many preoperative factors are the same as for any operation. They include the type and timing of skin preparation (shaving, etc.), increased time hospitalized before surgery, a concurrent distant infection, or recent surgery in the same operative field. Preoperative cardiopulmonary failure and requirement for an intra-aorta balloon pump increase the risk of postoperative infections as well.[16]

Patients who are taking steroids, have diabetes or a history of mediastinal radiation, or demonstrate mechanical abnormalities such as osteoporosis or pulmonary problems are at higher risk for the development of post–median sternotomy mediastinitis.

In a review from the Cleveland Clinic, the prevalence of wound complications in diabetics was 5.7% and in those without diabetes, 0.3% ($P = .01$). Age alone may be a significant variable. The incidence of infection in patients less than 60 years was 0.2%; this incidence increased to 1.6% in patients age 60 to 70 years and to 3.1% in those greater than 70 years of age. Women appear to have an increased risk for sternal wound problems.[1, 17] The higher incidence of osteoporosis as well as the distracting forces placed on the sternotomy by the weight of heavy breasts may lead to mechanical shear/stress and compromise operative repair in women. On the other hand, some reports indicate that males may have a increased risk of infection because of hirsutism.[16]

## Intra-operative Risk Factors

Operating rooms rarely contain more than 60 to 70 microorganisms per cubic foot in the air, a level far below the critical $10^5$ microorganisms that must lodge in tissue for infection to occur.[15] Studies of the operative environment have shown a startling number of positive cultures. The heart-lung machine demonstrates a positive culture in an astounding 71% of cases, whereas the patients themselves had multiple sites with positive cultures 20% of the time. Prosthetic valves were culture-positive in 50% of the patients, and the cardiotomy site was positive in 64%. However, clinical infection developed in only 2 of the 66 patients.[18] *Staphylococcus epidermidis* has been cultured from nasal cultures of 80% of operating room personnel. It has frequently been cultured from the inside of gloves and from 90% of wounds before closure, yet the incidence of clinical infection from this organism is still low.

Most studies show a higher incidence of sepsis with prolonged cardiopulmonary bypass (more than 3 hours).[19, 20] There is evidence that bypass affects phagocytic capacity. The ability to clear bacteria is diminished, a problem that increases with prolonged bypass time.[18]

Ulicny et al. examined the effect of acute-phase protein response (C-reactive protein, complement, etc.) and delayed hypersensitivity on the development of wound infection. Preoperative complement C3 levels were elevated in 80% of those with mediastinitis as compared with 30% of those with well-healed wounds. Postoperative $a_1$ acid glycoprotein levels were elevated in 80% of those with infection vs. 29% without infection. These apparent differences did not reach statistical significance.[21]

In addition to the duration of surgery, cardiopulmonary bypass time, and excessive bleeding, the use of one or two IMAs has been implicated as a risk factor associated with sternal infections. Kouchoukos et al. noted that sternal infections occurred with greater frequency in patients using both IMAs than among unilateral IMA or vein graft patients (6.9% vs. 1.9% vs. 1.3%, $P = .001$, n = 1,566 patients).[20] The Cleveland Clinic studies of relative risk as assessed by regression analysis revealed the combination of diabetes and bilateral IMA to have a relative risk of 5.00.[19] However, among conduit groups (saphenous vein, one IMA, or two IMAs), there was no difference. Hazelrigg et al. noted among 2,582 patients with a infection rate of 0.81% a significantly higher rate among those having bilateral IMA grafting (1.65%; odds ratio, 4.75).[22] The interaction of some preoperative and postoperative factors can be summarized in Figure 1. The presence of a conduit, obesity, and the duration of mechanical ventilation independently and collectively increase the risk of infection.[20]

There is a correlation between sternotomy technique and infection. The advent of high-speed mechanical devices has reduced infection rates as compared with Gigli (hand-driven) saws.[23] A pro-

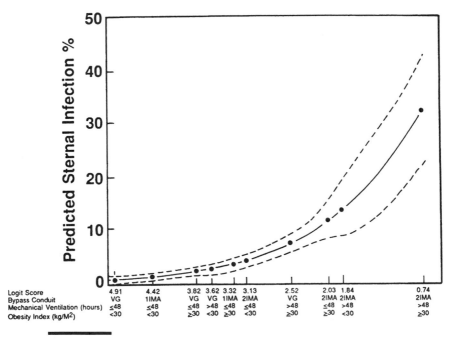

| Logit Score | 4.91 | 4.42 | 3.82 | 3.62 | 3.32 | 3.13 | 2.52 | 2.03 | 1.84 | 0.74 |
|---|---|---|---|---|---|---|---|---|---|---|
| Bypass Conduit | VG | 1IMA | VG | VG | 1IMA | 2IMA | VG | 2IMA | 2IMA | 2IMA |
| Mechanical Ventilation (hours) | ≤48 | ≤48 | ≤48 | >48 | ≤48 | ≤48 | >48 | ≤48 | >48 | >48 |
| Obesity Index (kg/M²) | <30 | <30 | ≥30 | <30 | ≥30 | <30 | ≥30 | ≥30 | <30 | ≥30 |

**FIGURE 1.**

Logit curve for the three independent predictors of sternal infection (bypass procedure, obesity index, and prolonged ventilation). *Broken lines* represent the standard error. (*VG* = vein grafts; *1 IMA* = one internal mammary artery; *2 IMA* = both internal mammary arteries. (From Kouchoukos NT, Wareing TH, Murphey SF, et al: *Ann Thorac Surg* 49:210–219, 1990. Used by permission.)

longed duration of surgery has a linear relationship with infection. Mediastinal infections are no exception. This is likely a reflection of the complexity and duration of potential lodgment of bacteria.[24]

Adequate sternal immobilization appears to have an impact on the incidence of post–median sternotomy mediastinitis. Osteoporosis, nonmidline sternotomies, transverse fractures of sternal segments, and severe pulmonary disease predispose to sternal instability. It is well accepted that stable bone healing and union depend on adequate reduction and immobilization of the bony fragments. To minimize inflammation and associated fluid collections as well as optimize osteosynthesis, rigid fixation principles should be employed.

The technique used to immobilize the sternum following median sternotomy has improved from nylon and silk sutures to more rigid approximation with wire. During the past two decades there have been several attempts to achieve fixation that is more rigid than that afforded with simple cerclage wires.[25–27] Sargent et al. demonstrated advanced sternal healing at 4 weeks after rigid fixation as compared with cerclage wire closure in a primate model.[28] We have reported successful healing with titanium miniplates in 29 patients: in 24 who were in secondary, closure after suppuration and in 5 treated preventively who were in high-risk groups.[29]

### Postoperative Risk Factors

Any major postoperative complication such as bleeding, impaired vascularity, and concurrent infection adds to the risk of post–median sternotomy mediastinitis. Bleeding and hematoma predispose to bacterial growth. Data confirm that operative bleeding contributes to mediastinitis. In one series, more than 53% of patients with mediastinitis had postoperative blood loss of more than 1,250 mL.[13] "Redo" or repeat surgery, either early or remote, is also a predisposing factor. Eighteen percent to 42% of patients with mediastinitis fit into this category.[12, 13] Similarly, postoperative shock or cardiopulmonary resuscitation increases complication rates two to four times.

As many as half of the patients with mediastinitis have had "low-flow" phenomena. Hypoperfusion states may cause decreased local host resistance to bacteria through compromised vascularity. Low cardiac output may also depress cellular immunity.

It is well accepted that individuals with infection elsewhere in the body are predisposed to mediastinal infection.[15] Patients with tracheotomies or those on prolonged mechanical ventilation are more susceptible to infection.[30] Intravenous catheters, urinary catheters, and other drainage tubes are portals for entry of microorganisms and may be sources for hematogenous seeding of operative sites.

## MICROBIOLOGY

The microorganisms causing infection most frequently are those indigenous to the patients and their environment. *Staphylococcus aureus* and *epidermidis* were the most common organisms isolated and in our recent review accounted for 42% of infections.[29] In Hazelrigg and colleagues' series, staphylococcal species were present in 11 of 15 cultures of wound infections.[22] In Grossi and associates' report, 56 of 77 patients with mediastinitis had gram-positive organisms in their wounds, 47 of which were staphylococcal species. Gram-negative organisms or mixed infections accounted for another 25% of infections.[11] However, on some infections no organisms can be recovered. The difficulty of culturing anaerobic organisms may lead to under-reporting of this group of bacteria.

Quantitative cultures of biopsy samples of contaminated or infected wounds are helpful diagnostically and therapeutically. In our series, 46% of the wounds contained more than $10^5$ microorganisms per gram of tissue. About a third of the patients had persistent levels above $10^5$ after debridement and require additional debridement before successful closure could be accomplished.[29]

## ANTIBACTERIALS

To be effective, an antibacterial agent must be chosen appropriately and administered in a timely fashion, in adequate doses, and by the proper route.[15] In surgical wounds, a timely manner dictates that to be delivered prophylactically, antibacterials be administered before or at least within the first several hours of wounding. Although systemic antibacterials may reach therapeutic tissue levels at the margin of well-vascularized tissue and prevent invasive wound sepsis, most surgical wound infections cannot be prevented by systemic antibacterial therapy instituted after closure. It is very difficult to achieve adequate tissue levels in wounds with systemic antibacterials.

Once an overt infection has developed and the wound is open, antibacterials are best delivered topically. The open sternotomy wound, the exposed mediastinum, and the granulating wound margins are biologically comparable to a burn wound, and lessons learned in burn therapy should be applied. Silver sulfadiazine and mafenide (Sulfamylon) are excellent antibacterials that penetrate well into granulating and infected tissue. On the other hand, povidone-iodine (Betadine)-soaked materials deliver an agent that although elegant for washing and skin decontamination, does not penetrate well into tissue. Many other agents can be delivered topically by constant or intermittent irrigation of the wound.

## DIAGNOSIS

Suppurative mediastinitis does not occur in the immediate postoperative period. Bacteria must first lodge in the wound and subsequently build to critical levels before infection is clinically manifested. Most causes of mediastinitis will begin to be apparent between 4 days and 3 weeks postoperatively. Prophylactic antibacterials, when used as part of the postoperative management, may actually delay the clinical appearance for 2 to 3 months.[18]

Purulent drainage through a wound is an obvious sign of infection. However, suspicion should be heightened in a patient whose pain begins to increase toward the end of the first postoperative week rather than decreasing and whose wounds become reddened and swollen. A high spiking fever will arouse suspicion and often heralds an abscess, yet a low-grade fever and leukocytosis should be carefully investigated because fever and leukocytosis are almost always present with mediastinitis. Patients in whom fever and leukocytosis develop must be suspected of harboring mediastinal sepsis, even if drainage has not appeared and the sternum clinically appears to be stable. Aspiration of the mediastinum is a straightforward diagnostic maneuver; it may be of low yield but is valuable when a positive culture results. Any drainage must be immediately cultured for both aerobic as well as anaerobic organisms, with determination of antibacterial sensitivity.[18]

Radiographic workup is limited. Routine chest films are neither sensitive nor specific. Computed tomographic scans may be helpful, particularly if gas-forming organisms are seen, but the sensitivity and specificity of these studies are suboptimal.

Patients who undergo cardiac surgery are often quite ill and may have a variety of concurrent infectious complications. Patients may experience infections in leg wounds (as high as 11.3%), infections in the urinary tract (4.6%), and pneumonia (2.5%).[30] One should not attribute systemic signs of infection to these sites and divert attention from the chest wound and thereby delay diagnosis.

## THERAPY

Sternal wound infections range from superficial to life-threatening mediastinitis (with or without osteomyelitis), and treatment must be tailored appropriately.

Suppurative mediastinitis is a surgical problem. Nonsurgical supportive care to respiratory, cardiovascular, and other systems is critical, and although systemic antibacterials are vital, they are strictly supportive and do not constitute definitive therapy. In a few patients, fever, leukocytosis, and other nonspecific signs may develop and then resolve with nonoperative measures. However, purulent drainage is an absolute indication for surgery, as is sternal instability.

The fundamental surgical approaches to any surgical infection include adequate debridement, proper cleansing, and the appropriate use of antibacterials.[15]

Debridement has the dual purpose of removing dead tissue and foreign body and helping to restore bacteriologic balance. The wound should be opened completely and suture material, wire, bone wax, and blood clots removed. Granulation tissue should be removed by sharp debridement or curettage from the wound edges, the cancellous bone of each sternal segment, as well as the surface of the heart. Biopsy samples from each of these ares should undergo routine quantitative tissue culture. Quantitative tissue cultures identify the type and quantity of organisms and provide antibacterial sensitivity within 18 to 24 hours (Fig 2, A).

Intraoperative irrigation should be performed under pressure. Large amounts of irrigation fluid are not nearly so important as mechanically removing the microorganisms and debris from the interstices of the soft tissue in which they are lodged. Pulsating jet lavage (7 psi) is as effective as a syringe with a fine needle directed to the wound. A bulb syringe is not adequate because it does not generate the necessary force to effectively remove the bacteria from the wound.

The bone is assessed clinically for vascularity (Fig 2, B). Exposed cartilage, devascularized bone, and bone found to have questionable vascularity should be removed. Experience and surgical judgment help determine the amount of tissue to be removed. Biopsy samples from the tissue remaining after debridement are submitted for intraoperative rapid slide quantitative bacteriologic analysis. The rapid slide technique allows a determination of bacterial content. If fewer than $10^5$ microorganisms per gram of tissue are present, closure may proceed safely[15] (Fig 2, C).

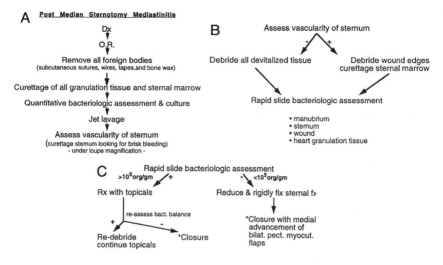

**A** Post Median Sternotomy Mediastinitis

Dx
↓
O.R.
↓
Remove all foreign bodies
(subcutaneous sutures, wires, tapes, and bone wax)
↓
Curettage of all granulation tissue and sternal marrow
↓
Quantitative bacteriologic assessment & culture
↓
Jet lavage
↓
Assess vascularity of sternum
(curettage sternum looking for brisk bleeding)
- under loupe magnification -

**B** Assess vascularity of sternum
- / +
Debride all devitalized tissue     Debride wound edges
curettage sternal marrow

Rapid slide bacteriologic assessment

• manubrium
• sternum
• wound
• heart granulation tissue

**C** Rapid slide bacteriologic assessment
>10⁵org/gm / +     - \ <10⁵org/gm
Rx with topicals     Reduce & rigidly fix sternal fx

re-assess bact. balance
+ / \ -
Re-debride     *Closure
continue topicals

*Closure with medial
advancement of
bilat. pect. myocut.
flaps

\*- Salvage of sternum &/or manubrium is dependent on vascularity
and bacteriologic control. If significant amount of sternum is removed,
remaining sternum &/or manubrium are reduced & rigidly fixed.
All remaining dead space is closed with muscle flaps.

---

**FIGURE 2.**

A–C, treatment algorithms.

The term *irrigation* has also been applied to a technique of postoperative management in which the contaminated but debrided wound is closed over irrigation catheters into which antibacterial or other irrigating solutions may be instilled. Catheters are used to collect the effluent with or without suction. Modern irrigating solutions include powerful antibiotics (polymyxin, bacitracin, etc.) not readily available for systemic use.[10, 31, 32] The use of closed-system drainage has been a very effective management technique when performed early.[2, 31] Introduced by Shumaker and Mandelbaum in 1963, it is a technique of value in lesser infections, particularly when large cavities ("dead space") are not a feature of the wound.[33] Debridement and closed irrigation were used successfully in 16 patients with hospitalization ranging from 18 to 44 days.[32] A more recent study comparing closed irrigation with other techniques found no difference in outcome.[10]

Although closed irrigation may suffice in some situations, experience over the past decade has taught us that it is difficult to determine which patients it will be efficacious. Therefore, to shorten hospital stay and allow the fewest interventions, we advocate initial debridement of all nonviable or infected bone and soft tissue, rigid fixation of the sternal segments that may be salvaged, and flap closure as needed.

## CLOSURE

Closure of the wound ideally involves two steps: reduction and fixation of retained viable sternum (if possible) and adequate soft tissue coverage. The timing of closure is dependent on bacterial control of the wound (Fig 2, C).

The thorax is both semirigid and flexible; removal of large segments of the sternum, costochondral areas, and ribs may be accomplished without major functional loss. Therefore, when bone is infected or marginally viable, it is far better to remove it. However, when the bone is healthy, the bony edges should be anatomically reduced and rigidly fixed. Rigid sternal fixation has been demonstrated to be safe and effective when quantitative counts in the retained, well-vascularized cancellous bone are less than $10^5$ organisms per gram.[29] Plate and screw fixation provides secure fixation even to very osteoporotic bone. This technique was used successfully in 24 patients with suppurative mediastinitis; 20 (83%) were closed in one operation, and 4 required two stages of debridement before closure.[29]

If all of the sternal bone is salvaged, then soft tissue closure is straightforward. There are theoretical and practical advantages to mobilizing the medial edges of the pectoralis major and rectus abdominis muscles on either side of the wound and advancing them to the midline. This maneuver provides an additional layer of tissue between the skin and the sternum. Separation of the pectoralis from its origin relieves tension from the sternal repair.

When a significant amount of sternal bone has been removed and the bony edges cannot be approximated, regional muscle provides closure of the defect and obliteration of potential "dead space" with well-vascularized tissue. It is usually possible to close the skin over the muscle flaps. Alternatively, each may be transferred as a myocutaneous unit if such a need arises. As final healing occurs, there is usually sufficient scarring to functionally stabilize the chest.

PECTORALIS MAJOR MUSCLE.—The pectoralis major muscle can be elevated by separating it from its origin, thus taking tension off the sternal repair. The freed muscle edges can be joined in the midline. When the humeral insertion is freed, the muscle is quite mobile and may be moved medially or turned over into cavitary defects. The pectoralis major is particularly valuable in the upper three fourths of the anterior mediastinum. Its arc of rotation is away from the xiphoid; thus its usefulness is limited in inferior defects. The wound surface is closed primarily or with skin grafts as necessary.

RECTUS ABDOMINIS MUSCLE.—A superiorly based rectus abdominis muscle may be transposed into the anterior mediastinum with or without a skin island. This flap has become the flap of choice for some. Although skin territories in patients who smoke or are obese may be unpredictable, the flap may even be used when the IMA has been employed by basing its blood supply on the intercostal vessels. Majure et al. have used the rectus flap on 14 patients and prefers this flap because of ease, dependability, and aesthetic considerations.[34] In the large series of Nahai et al., the rectus was used on 145 occasions with only a 3.3% complication rate.[23]

OMENTUM.—The omentum can be transposed to an extra-abdominal position. The omentum may be freed from the colon and rotated on either the left or the right gastroepiploic vessel. The extent of the area of rotation is adjustable by subdividing the vascularity and thus lengthening it.

The disadvantage of both the rectus abdominis muscle and omental flaps is the donor site. Abdominal wall incisions increase postoperative pain and may compromise respiratory function.

Open treatment is an alternative to immediate closure.[35] After debridement the wound is left open and treated with topical antibacterials. The progress of the treatment can be monitored with diagnostic precision by quantitative microbiologic techniques. Serial tissue biopsy studies are followed. When bacterial counts fall to less than $10^5$ bacteria per gram of tissue, bacteriologic balance has been achieved and the wound should be closed.[15, 29]

## RESULTS

Cheung et al.[4] compared the duration of hospital stay in patients treated for mediastinitis with two different techniques. The initial group of 8 patients was treated with debridement, closure, and tube irrigation. Subsequently, 16 patients were treated with debridement, partial sternal resection, and primary or delayed flap closure. Hospital stay averaged 365 days in the former group and 62 days in the later group.

Recently, Molina[36] has returned to the debridement, irrigation, primary closure routine reported by Shumaker and Mandelbaum[33] and later by Spencer's group.[32] Molina treated 16 cases of sternal infection associated with dehiscence. There was no major bone resection, two systems of tube irrigation were used (superficial and deep), and a Robicsek-type closure using vertical and circumferential wires was employed. No muscle flaps or skin advancement was added. Hospital stay was 14 to 18 days.

Most units have moved to debridement, bone resection, and primary closure with muscle flaps. We have recently reported a study of 24 patients treated over a 2½-year period at two institutions. Postoperative mediastinitis was treated with either complete or partial sternal salvage (based on clinical assessment of sternal vascularity and osseous bacteriologic assessment) and rigid internal fixation of the retained sternal segments. Twenty of 24 subjects were treated in one operation. Four patients were treated in a staged procedure in which debridement was followed by definitive closure after an interval of open wound care (1 to 7 days) required to achieve bacteriologic balance. Two patients had repairs complicated with early recurrent sternal instability and wound drainage and required additional debridement and closure with muscle flaps. All patients survived. The postoperative hospital stay ranged from 5 to 84 days with a mean of 17 and a median of 7 days.

## CONCLUSIONS

Suppurative mediastinitis is a modern problem, the consequence of extensive cardiac surgery. These patients are often ill before surgery, the surgery is often prolonged, and the "damaging effects" of cardiopulmonary bypass seem to predispose to infection.

The mortality from untreated suppurative mediastinitis is staggering, and no series can therefore include untreated controls. In one study, 73% of the patients died before early surgical intervention. The accuracy of diagnosis and the precision by which superficial infections are differentiated from sternal dehiscence or true suppurative mediastinitis are often unclear. In one large series, mediastinitis was diagnosed in 48 of 2,579 cases (1.86%).[3] Of these patients, 19 (40% of the infected cases but only 0.7% of all cases) died. It is difficult to compare the efficacy of "open" and "closed" techniques; certainly the more severe the infection, the more likely it would be that open treatment would be used. In another large series of 2,491 cases, suppurative mediastinitis developed in 36 patients (1.4%).[13] Twelve of these were considered to be high risk because of other non–infection-related problems, 10 of whom (83.3%) died. Of the remaining 24 patients, 8 were managed before techniques of debridement, open management, and flap closure were readily available, and 2 of these patients (25%) died. The subsequent 16 patients were managed by debridement, topical therapy, and flap closure, and 3 underwent valve replacement. Of these, only 1 (6%) in this most recent group died.

The standard treatment of post–median sternotomy mediastinitis has evolved over the past 35 years. Initially these infections were treated with debridement and the wound was left open and allowed to granulate and gradually close by secondary intention. This technique was associated with significant morbidity, mortality, and prolonged hospitalization.[23] In 1963, Schumaker and Mandelbaum[33] described the technique of closed catheter antibiotic irrigation following debridement and rewiring of the sternum. Thirteen years later, Lee et al.[37] treated those patients who failed catheter irrigation and rewiring with wide debridement followed by omental flap closure. Jurkiewicz and associates[38] expanded this concept by using muscle flaps to fill the dead space remaining after radical debridement. Although this approach is currently accepted as the treatment of choice for post–median sternotomy infections,[6, 39–42] it is not without significant long-term sequelae.[43]

We employed this standard approach beginning in the early 1980s. Uniformly, patients with postoperative mediastinitis had sternal instability with either loose, broken, or pulled-through wires. Often, a majority of the bone that was debrided and discarded appeared to be healthy with good vascularity. It was our belief that movement of the unstable sternum increases the inflammatory exudate, which in association with bone wax, residual hematoma, and other particulate matter, leads to infection. Thus we began attempting sternal salvage and employing the techniques of rigid fixation in 1990.

The principles of management of established mediastinitis include early diagnosis and prompt aggressive debridement. Salvage of the sternum and manubrium is dependent on its vascularity and bacteriologic control. The amount of bony debridement is primarily predicated on its vascularity. The appropriateness of wound closure is determined by quantitative bacteriologic assessment. Anatomic reduction and rigid internal fixation of the sternum should be performed when viable noninfected sternum is able to be preserved. Concerns of impeding emergent re-entry into the mediastinum are unfounded. A small plate cutter or heavy scissors can cut most miniplates, or they can easily be removed with a screw driver. Removal during delayed secondary operations is somewhat more difficult because of tissue adherence to titanium. In the future, this problem may be obviated by the use of absorbable plates.[44] If a large part of the sternum is removed, the remaining sternum is reduced and rigidly fixed. Muscle flaps are valuable in filling cavitary defects and obliterating dead space created from the sternal debridement. Closure may be performed immediately following debridement if one is assured that the wound is in bacteriologic balance, or closure may be delayed to allow a period of open treatment with topical antibacterials. Rewiring and continuous mediastinal antibiotic irrigation may be considered in early cases without suppuration. These techniques have seen a reduction in mortality from 73% to 100% with nonoperative management to less than 5% at present.

## REFERENCES

1. Grmoljez PF, Barner HH, Willman VL, et al: Major complications of median sternotomy. *Am J Surg* 130:679–681, 1975.
2. Breyer RH, Mills SA, Hudspeth AS, et al: A prospective study of sternal wound complications. *Ann Thorac Surg* 37:412–416, 1984.
3. Ottino G, De Paulis R, Pansini G, et al: Marjor sternal infection after open-heart surgery: A multivariate analysis of risk factors in 2,579 consecutive operative procedures. *Ann Thorac Surg* 44:173–179, 1987.
4. Cheung EH, Craver JM, Jones EL, et al: Mediastinitis after cardiac valve operations. *J Thorac Cardiovasc Surg* 90:517–522, 1985.
5. Pairolero PC, Arnold PG: Management of recalcitrant median sternotomy wounds. *J Thorac Cardiovasc Surg* 88:357–364, 1984.
6. Arnold PG, Pairolero PC: Chest wall reconstruction. *Ann Surg* 19:725–731, 1984.
7. Brown HA, Braimbridge MV, Panagopoulos P, et al: The complications of median sternotomy. *J Thorac Cardiovasc Surg* 58:189–196, 1969.
8. Miholic J, Hudec M, Domanig E, et al: Risk factors for severe bacterial infections after valve replacement and aortocoronary bypass operations: Analysis of 246 cases by logistic regression. *Ann Thorac Surg* 40:224–228, 1985.
9. Serry C, Bleck PC, Javid H, et al: Sternal wound complications. *J Thorac Cardiovasc Surg* 80:861–867, 1980.
10. Scully HE, Leclerc Y, Martin RD, et al: Comparison between antibiotic irrigation and mobilization of pectoralis muscle flaps in treatment of deep sternal infections. *J Thorac Cardiovasc Surg* 90:523–531, 1985.
11. Grossi EA, Culliford AT, Krieger KH, et al: A survey of 77 major infectious complications following median sternotomy: A review of 7,949 consecutive operative procedures. *Ann Thorac Surg* 40:214–223, 1985.
12. Rutledge R, Applebaum RE, Kim BJ: Mediastinal infection after open heart surgery. *Surgery* 97:88–92, 1985.
13. Culliford AT, Cunningham JN, Zeff RH, et al: Sternal and costochondral infections following open heart surgery. *J Thorac Cardiovasc Surg* 72:714–726, 1976.
14. Steigel RM, Beasley ME, Sink JD, et al: Management of postoperative

mediastinitis in infants and children by muscle flap rotation. *Ann Thorac Surg* 46:45, 1988.

15. Robson MC, Krizek TJ, Heggers JP: Biology of surgical infection, in Ravitch MM, Austen WG, Scott HW, et al (eds): *Current Problems in Surgery*. St Louis, Mosby, 1973, pp 1–62.
16. Demmy TL, Park SB, Liebler GA, et al: Recent experience with major sternal wound complications. *Ann Thorac Surg* 49:458–462, 1990.
17. Cosgrove DM, Lytle BW, Loop FD, et al: Does bilateral internal mammary artery grafting increase surgical risk? *J Thorac Cardiovasc Surg* 95:850–856, 1988.
18. Sarr MG, Gott VL, Townsend TR: Mediastinal infection after cardiac surgery. *Ann Thorac Surg* 38:415–423, 1984.
19. Loop FD, Lytle BW, Cosgrove DM, et al: Sternal wound complications after isolated coronary artery bypass grafting: Early and late mortality, morbidity, and cost of care. *Ann Thorac Surg* 49:179–187, 1990.
20. Kouchoukos NT, Wareing TH, Murphey SF, et al: Risk of bilateral internal mammary artery bypass grafting. *Ann Thorac Surg* 49:210–219, 1990.
21. Ulicny KS, Hiratzka LF, Williams RB, et al: Sternal infection: Poor prediction by acute phase response and delayed hypersensitivity. *Ann Thorac Surg* 50:949–958, 1990.
22. Hazelrigg SR, Wellons HA, Schneider JA, et al: Wound complications after median sternotomy. *J Thorac Cardiovasc Surg* 98:1096–1099, 1989.
23. Nahai F, Rand RP, Hester TR, et al: Primary treatment of the infected sternotomy wound with muscle flaps: A review of 211 cases. *Plast Reconstr Surg* 84:434–441, 1989.
24. Engelman RM, Williams CD, Gouge TH, et al: Mediastinitis following open-heart surgery. *Arch Surg* 107:772–778, 1973.
25. Hicks GL, Haake W, Stewart SS, et al: The nuts and bolts of sternal dehiscence. *Ann Thorac Surg* 36:364–365, 1983.
26. Miller MD, Johnson RG, Naifeh J: Repair of sternal dehiscence using a Harrington compression system. *Ann Thorac Surg* 45:684–685, 1988.
27. Al-Naaman YD, Al-Ani MS: Sternal staple: Simple and rapid device for closure of median sternotomy. *Ann Thorac Surg* 21:170–171, 1976.
28. Sargent LA, Seyfer AE, Hollinger J, et al: The healing sternum; a comparison of osseous healing with wire vs. rigid fixation. *Ann Thorac Surg* 52:490–494, 1991.
29. Gottlieb LJ, Pielet RW, Karp RP, et al: Rigid internal fixation of the sternum in post-operative mediastinitis. *Arch Surg* 129:489–493, 1994.
30. Verkkala K: Occurrence of and microbiological findings in postoperative infections following open-heart surgery. *Ann Clin Res* 19:170–177, 1987.

31. Acinpura AJ, Godfrey N, Romita M, et al: Surgical management of infected median sternotomy: Closed irrigation vs. muscle flaps. *J Cardiovasc Surg* 26:443–446, 1985.

32. Bryant LR, Spencer FC, Trinkle JK: Treatment of median sternotomy infection by mediastinal irrigation with an antibiotic solution. *Surgery* 169:914–920, 1969.

33. Schumacker HB, Mandelbaum I: Continuous antibiotic irrigation in the treatment of infection. *Arch Surg* 86:384–387, 1963.

34. Majure JA, Albin RE, O'Donnell RS, et al: Reconstruction of the infected median sternotomy wound. *Ann Thorac Surg* 42:9–12, 1986.

35. Fanning WJ, Vasko JS, Kilman JW: Delayed sternal closure after cardiac surgery. *Ann Thorac Surg* 44:169–172, 1987.

36. Molina JE: Primary closure for infected dehiscence of the sternum. *Ann Thorac Surg* 55:459–463, 1993.

37. Lee AB, Schimert G, Shatkin S: Total excision of the sternum and thoracic pedicle transposition of the greater omentum. *Surgery* 80:433–436, 1976.

38. Jurkiewicz MJ, Bostwick J, Hester TR, et al: Infected median sternotomy wound: Successful treatment with muscle flaps. *Ann Surg* 191:738–744, 1980.

39. Arnold PG, Pairolero PC: The use of pectoralis major muscle flaps to repair defects of the anterior chest wall. *Plast Reconstr Surg* 63:205–213, 1979.

40. Nahai F, Morales L, Bone DK, et al: Pectoralis major muscle turnover flaps for the closure of infected sternotomy wound with preservation of form and function. *Plast Reconstr Surg* 70:471–474, 1982.

41. Herrera HR, Ginsburg ME: The pectoralis major myocutaneous flap and omental transposition for closure of infected median sternotomy wounds. *Plast Reconstr Surg* 70:465–470, 1982.

42. Seguin JR, Loisance DY: Omental transposition for closure of median sternotomy following severe mediastinal and vascular infection. *Chest* 80:684–686, 1985.

43. Ringelman PR, Vander Kolk CA, Cameron D, et al: Long term results of flap reconstruction in median sternotomy wound infections. *Plast Reconstr Surg* 96:1208–1214, 1994.

44. Matsui T, Kitano M, Nakamura T, et al: Bioabsorbable struts made from poly-L-lactide and their application for treatment of chest deformity. *J Thorac Cardiovasc Surg* 108:162–168, 1994.

# The Use of Positron Emission Tomography Imaging in the Management of Patients With Ischemic Cardiomyopathy

**Jamshid Maddahi, M.D.**
Division of Nuclear Medicine and Biophysics, Department of Molecular and Medical Pharmacology, UCLA School of Medicine, Los Angeles, California

**Arie Blitz, M.D.**
Division of Cardiothoracic Surgery, Department of Surgery, UCLA School of Medicine, Los Angeles, California

**Michael Phelps, Ph.D.**
Division of Nuclear Medicine and Biophysics, Department of Molecular and Medical Pharmacology, UCLA School of Medicine, Los Angles, California

**Hillel Laks, M.D.**
Division of Cardiothoracic Surgery, Department of Surgery, UCLA School of Medicine, Los Angeles, California

---

C oronary artery disease (CAD) is the most common cause of heart failure in the United States. According to the National Heart, Lung, and Blood Institute, there are 400,000 new cases of heart failure and over 200,000 deaths from heart failure each year. Currently, over 2 million Americans have heart failure. In addition, ischemic cardiomyopathy, which has a major overlapping group of patients in congestive heart failure, accounts for approximately 40% to 50% of the patients referred for heart transplantation in the United States. Hence the management of these patients has become an important focus of the health care industry.

## MANAGEMENT OPTIONS FOR PATIENTS WITH ISCHEMIC CARDIOMYOPATHY

The management algorithm for patients with ischemic cardiomyopathy is both controversial and evolving. Before the advent of imaging techniques to determine myocardial viability, many patients with CAD and low ejection fractions were relegated to medical therapy. Yet medical therapy has been associated with mortality rates ranging from 15% to 60% per year.[1-18] Table 1 lists published results on the characteristics and actuarial survival of medically treated patients with ischemic cardiomyopathy.[3, 5, 10, 13-19] A problem arises in attempting to compare the results from different clinical studies inasmuch as ischemic cardiomyopathy is variably defined in the literature.

Although authors generally equate ischemic cardiomyopathy with the presence of angiographically demonstrable CAD and reduced ventricular function, the latter is often gauged in different fashions, e.g., by ejection fraction, the number of dyskinetic segments, or the degree of congestive heart failure. In addition, the cutoff used for some of these indices may also vary from study to study. For the purposes of compiling a literature review, we have restricted the term *ischemic cardiomyopathy* to those studies including only patients with a left ventricular ejection fraction (LVEF) of less than or equal to 40% regardless of the patient's symptom status. Studies including patients with higher ejection fractions are thus not included in this analysis. At UCLA Medical Center we use a somewhat more stringent criterion and set the ejection fraction cutoff at less than or equal to 30%.

From the studies listed in Table 1 it is evident that in addition to a variable ejection fraction cutoff ranging from 20% to 40%, the symptom status of the patient is also quite variable across studies. Angina was present in 37% to 100% (mean, 69% ± 25%) of the patients, and symptoms of congestive heart failure were present in 19% to 55% (mean, 35% ± 16%). Mean 1-year and 5-year actuarial survival rates were 74% (range, 52% to 89%) and 44% (range, 18% to 60%), respectively. Thus there is a substantial mortality rate for patients with ischemic cardiomyopathy who are treated medically, particularly in studies including higher percentages of patients with congestive heart failure.[9] In addition, there is a trend in the more recent studies (i.e., after 1984) for an increasing prominence of congestive failure and a decreasing prominence of angina as a clinical feature.

During the 1980s, heart transplantation emerged as an impor-

**TABLE 1.**
Actuarial Survival of Patients With Ischemic Cardiomyopathy Undergoing Medical Management

| Author | Year | N | EF,* % | Inclusion of Patients With Aneurysm, Yes/No | Angina, % | CHF, % | Actuarial Survival (%) by Years of Follow-Up | | | | | | |
|---|---|---|---|---|---|---|---|---|---|---|---|---|---|
| | | | | | | | 1 | 2 | 3 | 4 | 5 | 6 | 7 |
| Yatteau[3] | 1974 | 42 | ≤25 | Y | 76 | 50 | 60 | 55 | | | | | |
| Manley[5] | 1976 | 63 | <20 | N | 100 | N/A | 52 | 31 | 25 | 23 | 18 | 10 | |
| Faulkner[7] | 1977 | 70 | ≤30 | N | 74 | 26 | 78 | 47 | 39 | 7 | | | |
| Alderman[10] | 1983 | 420 | ≤35 | Y | 56 | 19 | 84 | 74 | 65 | 61 | 53 | 45 | |
| Mock[13] | 1982 | 909 | <35 | N/A | N/A | N/A | | | | 58 | 52 | | |
| Pigott[14] | 1985 | 115 | ≤35 | N | 37 | 26 | 70 | 62 | 55 | 53 | 45 | 39 | 34 |
| Bounous[15] | 1988 | 409 | ≤40 | Y | N/A | N/A | 89 | 78 | 71 | 65 | 60 | 55 | 52 |
| Califf[17] | 1989 | 5,809 | ≤35 | N | 100 | N/A | 82 | 75 | 64 | 60 | 53 | 49 | 43 |
| Luciani[18] | 1993 | 72 | <30 | N | 43 | 55 | 74 | 60 | 50 | 42 | 28 | | |

*EF = ejection fraction; CHF = congestive heart failure; N/A = not available.

tant therapeutic alternative for patients with ischemic cardiomyopathy. However, as transplant waiting lists and waiting times have
progressively lengthened, up to a third of the patients listed for
transplantation die while waiting.[20] Table 2 lists the United Network for Organ Sharing (UNOS) data for cardiac transplantation
during the period of 1988 to 1994. As can be seen from the table,
the number of transplants has increased by about 40%, but most of
this increase occurred before 1990 and very little increase has been
seen since then. In addition, the number of patients remaining on
the waiting list at year's end has increased by over 180%, and the
number of patients dying while on the waiting list has increased
by 48%. Furthermore, median waiting periods have increased by
over 92%. Hence despite an initial increase in the number of heart
transplants performed in the late 1980s, this number has since sta-
bilized and more patients are dying while awaiting transplantation.
These trends have provided the impetus for a re-examination of
revascularization as a treatment alternative for patients with ischemic cardiomyopathy.

It has become well established that the long-term benefit of revascularization in patients with low ejection fractions is superior
to that of medical therapy. Nonetheless, during the early years of
revascularization surgery, the operative mortality in this group of
patients had been reported to be as high as 50%. Thus despite superior long-term results in operative survivors, the high opera-

**TABLE 2.**

United Network for Organ Sharing Heart Transplantation Data
1988–1994

| Year | Number Actually Transplanted | Number on Waiting List at Year's End | Median Waiting Period, Days | Number Died Waiting |
|------|------|------|------|------|
| 1988 | 1,675 | 1,030 | 108 | 492 |
| 1989 | 1,705 | 1,320 | 128 | 519 |
| 1990 | 2,107 | 1,788 | 156 | 611 |
| 1991 | 2,125 | 2,267 | 197 | 779 |
| 1992 | 2,171 | 2,690 | 245 | 774 |
| 1993 | 2,298 | 2,834 | 208 | 762 |
| 1994 | 2,340 | 2,933 | N/A* | 730 |

*N/A = not available.

tive mortality rate in these patients had daunted many surgeons from performing bypass surgery in the past.[21, 22] Yet with recent improvements in anesthetic induction, myocardial protection, completeness of revascularization, and perioperative patient management, the operative mortality rate has been reduced to as low as 0% in one series,[23] and the majority of other series have reported operative mortality rates of less than 10%.[7, 10, 23–29] Improvements in myocardial protection have included cold potassium cardioplegia, warm blood induction cardioplegia, and retrograde coronary perfusion. Perioperative care has been optimized by the increased use of hemodynamic monitoring devices, intra-aortic balloon pumps, and ventricular assist devices.

A review of the surgical mortality statistics in the literature on ischemic cardiomyopathy reveals a wide range of operative mortality and long-term survival rates (Table 3).* These studies are difficult to compare for several reasons. First, as mentioned before, authors vary in their definition of ischemic cardiomyopathy. A variety of ejection fraction criteria have been used, some studies liberally including patients with ejection fractions below 40%,[15, 28] whereas others more stringently maintain a cutoff of 20%.[26] Second, studies report on different clinical subgroups of patients. Some report on all patients operated on below a certain ejection fraction,[10–12, 15, 25, 28, 34] and others restrict their results to patients with angina[23, 29, 31, 33, 35] or patients with congestive heart failure.[36] Still others report results that include patients who have undergone emergent revascularization for unstable angina, evolving myocardial infarction, or cardiogenic shock[16, 19, 26, 32] or patients who have undergone concomitant procedures (e.g., left ventricular aneurysmectomy, mitral valve replacement).[31]

Despite these conflicting results, it is clear from the data that revascularization can be performed with low operative mortality and excellent long-term survival in many centers. Table 3 lists a review of the published data on patient characteristics and survival after revascularization for ischemic cardiomyopathy. If we restrict analysis to series published during the most recent decade of cardiac surgery (i.e., 1984 to 1994), the mean operative mortality rate was 6.8%, ranging from 0% to 16%. The mean actuarial survival rates at 1 and 5 years were 86% ± 7% and 76% ± 11%, respectively.

Before the development of cardiac imaging techniques, the decision as to which patients with ischemic cardiomyopathy might

---

*References 3, 5, 7, 10, 14–16, 19, 23–33.

**TABLE 3.**
Characteristics, Hospital Mortality, and Actuarial Survival of Patients Undergoing Revascularization for Ischemic Cardiomyopathy

| Author | Year | N | EF, %* | Inclusion of Patients With Aneurysmectomy, Yes/No | Inclusion of Patients With Shock, Unstable Angina, or Acute MI Yes/No |
|---|---|---|---|---|---|
| Yatteau[3] | 1974 | 24 | ≤25 | Y | N |
| Mitchel[30] | 1975 | 40 | <40 | N | N |
| Manley[5] | 1976 | 246 | <31 | N | N/A |
| Faulkner[7] | 1977 | 46 | ≤30 | N | Y |
| Hung[31] | 1980 | 25 | ≤35 | N | N/A |
| Coles[29] | 1981 | 59 | m 28 | N | N/A |
| Alderman[10] | 1983 | 231 | <35 | Y | N/A |
| Hochberg (a)†[32] | 1983 | 425 | 20–39 | N | Y |
| Hochberg (b)[32] | 1983 | 41 | <20 | N | Y |
| Freeman[23] | 1984 | 18 | <40 | N | N/A |
| Tyras[28] | 1984 | 107 | <40 | N | N/A |
| Pigott[14] | 1985 | 77 | ≤35 | N | Y |
| Bounous[15] | 1988 | 301 | <40 | Y | N |
| Kron[27] | 1989 | 39 | ≤20 | N | N |
| Louie[33] | 1991 | 19 | m 23 | N | N |
| Christakis (a)[26] | 1992 | 2,539 | 20–40 | N | Y |
| Christakis (b)[26] | 1992 | 487 | ≤20 | N | Y |
| Luciani[19] | 1993 | 49 | <30 | N/A | Y |
| Van Trigt[16] | 1993 | 118 | ≤25 | N/A | Y |
| Elefteriades[25] | 1993 | 83 | ≤30 | N | Y |
| Dreyfus[24] | 1994 | 46 | m 23 | N | N/A |

*EF = ejection fraction; CHF = congestive heart failure; N/A = not available; MI = myocardial infarction; m = only mean ejection fraction available.
†Letters in parentheses refer to discrete subgroups of patients for the respective study.

| Angina, % | CHF, % | Hospital Mortality, % | Actuarial Survival (%) by Years of Follow-Up | | | | | | |
|---|---|---|---|---|---|---|---|---|---|
| | | | 1 | 2 | 3 | 4 | 5 | 6 | 7 |
| N/A | N/A | 33 | 45 | 40 | | | | | |
| 95 | 42 | 20 | N/A | N/A | N/A | N/A | N/A | N/A | N/A |
| 100 | 56 | 9–25 | 80 | 78 | 75 | 68 | 60 | 58 | |
| 100 | 43 | 4 | 95 | 83 | 78 | 78 | | | |
| 100 | 72 | 12 | 83 | 73 | 73 | | | | |
| 100 | 20 | 1.7 | 91 | 90 | 89 | 85 | 80 | | |
| 76 | 10 | 6.9 | 90 | 84 | 78 | 72 | 69 | 66 | |
| 100 | N/A | 11 | 80 | 72 | 60 | | | | |
| 100 | N/A | 37 | 38 | 23 | 15 | | | | |
| 100 | 100 | 0 | N/A | N/A | N/A | N/A | N/A | N/A | N/A |
| 94 | 31 | 3.7 | 91 | 89 | 89 | 89 | 89 | | |
| 65 | 21 | 1.3 | 94 | 88 | 83 | 82 | 76 | 70 | 63 |
| N/A | N/A | N/A | 89 | 88 | 84 | 82 | 80 | 75 | 75 |
| 56 | 67 | 2.6 | 88 | 83 | 83 | | | | |
| 23 | 100 | 16 | 72 | 72 | 72 | | | | |
| 100 | N/A | 4.8 | N/A | N/A | N/A | N/A | N/A | N/A | N/A |
| 100 | N/A | 9.8 | N/A | N/A | N/A | N/A | N/A | N/A | N/A |
| 67 | 23 | 14 | 85 | 83 | 83 | 79 | 79 | | |
| 100 | 65 | 11 | 77 | 68 | 65 | 60 | 58 | | |
| 49 | 52 | 8.4 | 87 | 87 | 80 | | | | |
| N/A | 100 | 2.2 | 87 | 87 | | | | | |

benefit from revascularization was a difficult one. Initial studies revealed that patients who had angina as their predominant symptom had a better outcome than those patients who had congestive heart failure. The presence of angina has been taken to imply the existence of viable but jeopardized myocardium, which in turn has implied the potential for a therapeutic benefit from revascularization. The absence of angina, however, has not necessarily implied a poorer outcome.[27] Therefore, a clear need has emerged for the development of techniques to ascertain which patients with ischemic cardiomyopathy would be appropriate candidates for revascularization. Although the diagnostic techniques conventionally used in the preoperative assessment of these patients allow one to assess coronary artery anatomy and disease as well as wall motion and ejection fraction, they fall short in giving us useful information concerning the reversibility of dysfunctioning myocardial segments.

The key to detecting reversibility in these segments centers on the concept of "hibernating myocardium" introduced by Rahimtoola.[37] Hibernating myocardium is myocardium that harbors viable tissue that has been "downregulated" by chronic ischemia so that myocardial energy demands do not outstrip myocardial energy supply (see later). Hence such myocardium has perfusion that is sufficient to maintain viability but insufficient for normal myocardial function. This is in contradistinction to infarcted tissue, where an inadequate blood supply has rendered the tissue infarcted and scarred. The implication of the existence of hibernating myocardium is thus clear: revascularization of hibernating segments should improve myocardial function. This concept has provided the springboard for the development of techniques like cardiac positron emission tomography (PET) for distinguishing viable hibernating myocardium from scarred myocardium.

## BASIS FOR THE USE OF POSITRON EMISSION TOMOGRAPHY METABOLIC TRACERS TO ASSESS MYOCARDIAL VIABILITY

In patients with CAD, left ventricular contractile dysfunction (dyssynergy) may be due to (1) transmural myocardial infarction, (2) nontransmural myocardial infarction, (3) myocardial hibernation, or (4) myocardial stunning, which are different from one another with respect to the potential for recovery of dyssynergy after myocardial revascularization. In transmural myocardial infarction, myocardial necrosis involves the full thickness of the myocardium, whereas in nontransmural myocardial infarction, myocardial necrosis is either limited to the subendocardium or is scattered throughout the myocardium. Revascularization is not expected to improve left ventricular dyssynergy in these two conditions. The term *hibernating myocardium* was coined by Dr. Rahimtoola[37, 38] to define abnormal left ventricular function at rest that is due to chronic painless, persistent severe "ischemia" at rest and that is reversible. Hibernating myocardium is a result of reduced myocardial blood flow that causes decreased myocardial contractility while viability is maintained. Restoration of normal blood flow to hibernating myocardium is expected to reverse contractile dysfunction. Myocardial stunning results from periods of severe ischemia that are too brief to cause myocardial necrosis and may nonetheless be associated with ultrastructural and biochemical changes and, most importantly, with contractile dysfunction that persists for prolonged periods after restoration of perfusion.[39] This situation is observed clinically when reperfusion is induced after coronary occlusion and salvages some of the jeopardized tissue. The return of contractile function in the salvaged tissue is generally not immediate and may require weeks to months.

With PET, positron-emitting radionuclides are used to obtain tomographic images of regional myocardial perfusion, metabolism, and receptor density. Four different PET approaches have been used for assessment of myocardial viability: (1) perfusion–[$^{18}$F]2-fluoro-2-deoxyglucose-(FDG) metabolism imaging, (2) determination of oxidative metabolism with $^{11}$C acetate, (3) uptake and retention of $^{82}$Rb, and (4) the water perfusable tissue index. By far, myocardial viability has been more extensively evaluated with the myocardial perfusion–FDG metabolism PET method than with other PET protocols. Therefore, the myocardial perfusion–FDG metabolism PET protocol will be the main focus of this chapter. With this protocol, regional myocardial perfusion is first evaluated with $^{13}$N ammonia, $^{82}$Rb, or $^{15}$O water. Subsequently, FDG is used to assess regional glucose utilization. Regional myocardial distribution of all the three PET perfusion tracers has been shown to be related to regional myocardial blood flow and the extraction fraction of the myocardium for a given tracer, which has been well characterized.[40–46] These tracers, however, have different imaging characteristics; the physical half-life of $^{13}$N ammonia is relatively longer (10 minutes) than that of $^{82}$Rb (75 seconds) and $^{15}$O water (2 minutes), thus allowing a longer imaging time and higher image count density with $^{13}$N ammonia. Since $^{15}$O water is rapidly exchanged between blood and surrounding tissue, blood pool subtraction techniques are needed to delineate myocardial uptake of [15]O water, further complicating the clinical imaging protocol and reducing [15]O water myocardial image quality. [13]N ammonia and [15]O water are cyclotron produced, whereas [82]Rb may be produced by a portable generator.

A glucose analogue, FDG, crosses the capillary and sarcolemmal membrane at a rate proportionate to that of glucose. After myocardial uptake, FDG is phosphorylated to FDG-6-phosphate and is then trapped in the myocardium because unlike phosphorylated glucose, it is a poor substrate for glycogen synthesis, the fructose phosphate shunt, and glycolysis.[47, 48] Regional myocardial uptake of FDG therefore reflects the relative distribution of regional rates

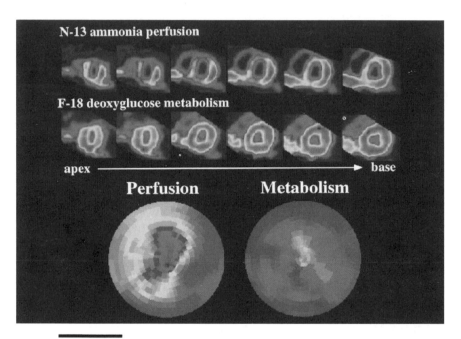

**FIGURE 1.**

PET images of a patient with ischemic cardiomyopathy that demonstrate the PET perfusion-metabolism mismatch pattern. The short axis N-13 ammonia perfusion PET images show severe hypoperfusion of the anterior, septal, and inferoseptal regions of the left ventricle. The corresponding short axis F-18 deoxyglucose (FDG) metabolism PET images show normal FDG uptake in the hypoperfused regions (i.e., perfusion-metabolism mismatch pattern). The polar map diplays (lower row) are derived from quantitation of activity in the entire left ventricle and confirm the mismatch pattern.

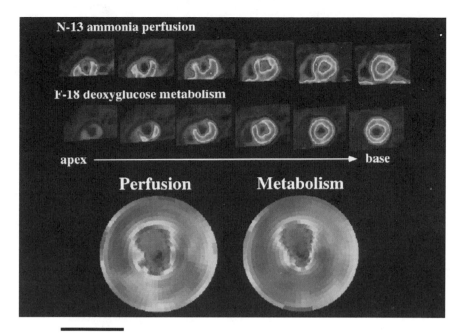

**FIGURE 2.**

PET images of a patient with ischemic cardiomyopathy that demonstrates the PET perfusion-metabolism match pattern. The short axis and polar map images show severe hypoperfusion and hypometabolism of the inferior region of the left ventricle (i.e., perfusion-metabolism match pattern).

of exogenous glucose utilization.[47-50] In the fasting state, fatty acids are the preferred myocardial substrate for adenosine triphosphate (ATP) production, and FDG is taken up very little if any by the myocardium.[50, 51] In ischemic myocardial regions, however, regional substrate utilization shifts from fatty acid oxidation to glucose utilization.[52-54] Hibernating myocardium would therefore demonstrate increased FDG uptake in the fasting state, unlike the surrounding normal myocardium. In the postprandial state, normal myocardium shifts from fatty acid to glucose as the primary substrate for ATP production; thus hibernating and normal myocardium would both demonstrate FDG uptake. Therefore, preserved or even enhanced FDG uptake in dysfunctional myocardial regions represents the presence of myocardial viability. It is possible that membrane-related ATP that is glycolytically derived is essential for cell survival (i.e., maintenance of transmembrane ion concentration gradients), which may indeed account for the enhanced FDG uptake.[55]

With the PET perfusion-metabolism protocol, when FDG is injected in the postprandial state, three different patterns of myocardial viability may be observed (Figs 1 and 2). Regional myocardial perfusion and FDG uptake may be concordantly reduced or absent, the so-called perfusion metabolism match pattern. Based on the severity of perfusion and FDG deficit, the "match" pattern may be categorized as a transmural match (absent or markedly reduced perfusion and FDG uptake) or a nontransmural match (mildly to moderately reduced perfusion and FDG uptake). We have used these two terms to indicate that transmural match implies the presence of transmural myocardial infarction and nontransmural match suggests the presence of a mixture of viable and nonviable tissue in a given myocardial region and thus nontransmural myocardial necrosis. When regional myocardial FDG uptake is disproportionately enhanced as compared with regional myocardial blood flow, the pattern is termed perfusion-metabolism "mismatch." This PET pattern is thought to represent hibernating myocardium. Regional dysfunction caused by myocardial stunning may be manifested by normal blood flow and normal, enhanced, or reduced glucose utilization.

## PREDICTION OF POSTREVASCULARIZATION RECOVERY OF REGIONAL LEFT VENTRICULAR DYSFUNCTION BY POSITRON EMISSION TOMOGRAPHY

Table 4 summarizes the results from 8 studies that have reported the value of myocardial perfusion–FDG metabolism match and mismatch patterns for predicting postrevascularization improvement of regional left ventricular contractile dysfunction.[56–63] A total of 396 dyssynergic myocardial segments were reported in 144 patients. The average reported positive and negative predictive accuracies for the PET mismatch pattern were 83% (209/251) and 83% (121/145), respectively. The positive predictive accuracies ranged from 72% to 95%, and the negative predictive accuracies ranged from 75% to 100%. In three studies,[56, 58, 59] FDG uptake was assessed in the fasting state, whereas the remaining five studies[57, 60–63] evaluated regional myocardial FDG uptake in the glucose-loaded state. Theoretically, fasting FDG studies may demonstrate small but functionally insignificant amounts of hibernating myocardium because of low myocardial background activity (no FDG uptake by the surrounding normal and nonviable myocardial segments). Although this has been thought to diminish the positive predictive accuracy of fasting FDG studies for recovery of

**TABLE 4.**

Predictive Accuracies of Perfusion–FDG* Metabolism PET Imaging for Recovery of Regional Left Ventricular Dyssynergy After Myocardial Revascularization

| | | Predictive Accuracy | |
|---|---|---|---|
| Author | N (Segs)† | Positive | Negative |
| Tillisch,[57] 1986 | 17 (67) | 35/41 (85%) | 24/26 (92%) |
| Tamaki,[58] 1989 | 20 (46) | 18/23 (78%) | 18/23 (78%) |
| Tamaki,[56] 1991 | 11 (56) | 40/50 (80%) | 6/6 (100%) |
| Lucignani,[59] 1992‡ | 14 (54) | 37/39 (95%) | 12/15 (80%) |
| Carrel,[60] 1992 | 23 (23) | 16/19 (84%) | 3/4 (75%) |
| Gropler,[61] 1992 | 16 (53) | 19/24 (79%) | 24/29 (83%) |
| Gropler,[62] 1993 | 34 (57) | 21/29 (72%) | 23/28 (82%) |
| Paolini,[63] 1994‡ | 9 (40) | 23/26 (88%) | 11/14 (79%) |
| Total | 144 (396) | 209/251 (83%) | 121/145 (83%) |

*FDG = [18F]2-fluoro-2-deoxyglycose; PET = positron emission tomography.
†Number of dyssynergic myocardial segments.
‡Hybrid imaging method using 99mTc-sestamibi single proton emission computed tomography and FDG PET.

regional left ventricular dysfunction, the average reported positive predictive accuracy for fasting FDG studies is 85% and appears to be similar to the average positive predictive accuracy of FDG studies after glucose loading, which is 81%. Different approaches to analysis of the perfusion and metabolism pattern, however, may affect the predictive accuracy. Gropler et al.[62] first normalized the relative uptake of perfusion tracer and FDG to their respective highest tracer activity concentrations and then evaluated ratios of FDG to the perfusion image as criteria for match and mismatch. This approach differs from the original one that normalized the myocardial FDG uptake to the myocardial region with the highest perfusion (upper 10% of the tracer concentration) and defined match and mismatch by differences between FDG and perfusion rather than ratios. The "ratio" approach had an even lower positive predictive accuracy (52%) when myocardial segments with milder degrees of regional contractile dysfunction were included in the analysis.

In one study,[64] FDG was injected after exercise rather than at rest in 16 patients. The reported positive and negative predictive accuracies with this approach were 68% and 79%, respectively. As with reversible exercise [201]Tl defects, postexercise myocardial uptake of FDG is expected to be observed in regions with exercise-induced ischemia as well as hibernating myocardium, thus resulting in a lower positive predictive accuracy for recovery of left ventricular dysfunction. In another study,[65] regional FDG uptake, without comparison to perfusion, was used to predict recovery of regional myocardial dyssynergy. These investigators performed receiver operating curve analysis of various thresholds for normalized regional FDG uptake and determined that an 85% to 90% value yielded a sensitivity of 85% and a specificity of 84% for the detection of regional functional recovery after revascularization. Reanalysis of these data shows that this threshold is associated with a positive predictive accuracy of 70% (23/33) and a negative predictive accuracy of 93% (53/57) for prediction of functional recovery after revascularization. It should be noted that without comparing regional FDG uptake with regional myocardial perfusion, it would not be possible to determine whether myocardial perfusion is concordantly reduced (nontransmural match pattern) or myocardial perfusion is more severely reduced (mismatch pattern). As stated earlier, such a distinction is important because the former is not expected to demonstrate recovery after myocardial revascularization. In studies by Lucignani et al.[59] and Paolini et al.[63] and a preliminary report from vom Dahl et al.,[66] a "hybrid" imaging approach was used in which myocardial perfusion was assessed by [99m]Tc-sestamibi single proton emission computed tomography (SPECT) and myocardial metabolism was evaluated by FDG PET imaging. The positive and negative predictive accuracies of the hybrid imaging method for postrevascularization recovery of regional left ventricular dysfunction were similar to those reported for the standard PET technique.

## PREDICTION OF POSTREVASCULARIZATION RECOVERY OF GLOBAL LEFT VENTRICULAR FUNCTION BY POSITRON EMISSION TOMOGRAPHY

Literature reports on the value of PET for predicting improvement in LVEF are predominantly presented as a comparison between prerevascularization and postrevascularization LVEFs in patients with and those without a significant perfusion–FDG metabolism mismatch. The results are summarized in Table 5 for three studies.[57, 67, 68] In all five studies,[57, 59, 63, 67, 68] the average LVEF significantly increased from before to after revascularization in patients who had the PET pattern of perfusion-metabolism mismatch. In

**TABLE 5.**
Value of Perfusion-Metabolism Positron Emission Tomography Studies for Predicting Improvement in Left Ventricular Ejection Fraction After Myocardial Revascularization

| Author | N | Patients With Mismatch | | Patients Without Mismatch | |
|--------|---|------|------|------|------|
|        |   | Pre* | Post | Pre | Post |
| Tillisch,[57] 1986 | 17 | 30 ± 11 | 45 ± 14 | 30 ± 11 | 31 ± 12 |
| Besozzi,[67] 1992 | 56 | 29 ± 12 | 41 ± 11 | 43 ± 10 | 39 ± 16 |
| Depre,[68] 1993† | 23 | 43 ± 18 | 52 ± 15 | 35 ± 9 | 24 ± 8 |
| Lucignani,[59] 1992‡ | 14 | 38 ± 5 | 48 ± 4 | — | — |
| Paolini,[63] 1994‡ | 17 | 28 ± 5 | 43 ± 8 | — | — |

*Pre = prerevascularization; Post = postrevascularization.
†Left ventricular ejection fraction data are not part of the published abstract but were presented at the 1993 American Heart Association meeting.
‡Hybrid imaging method using $^{99m}$Tc-sestamibi single proton emission computed tomography and fluorodeoxyglucose positron emission tomography.

three of five studies[57, 67, 68] in which LVEF was also determined, LVEF remained unchanged or decreased following revascularization in patients who did not have the PET pattern of perfusion-metabolism mismatch.

## PREDICTION OF POSTREVASCULARIZATION IMPROVEMENT IN HEART FAILURE BY POSITRON EMISSION TOMOGRAPHY

Because most patients with poor left ventricular function have heart failure symptoms, an important goal in assessing myocardial viability is to predict recovery of heart failure symptoms following myocardial revascularization. This question has been addressed by two groups of investigators using myocardial perfusion–FDG metabolism PET imaging. Eitzman and colleagues[69] used PET to assess myocardial viability in 82 patients with poor left ventricular function (average LVEF, 34%). Improvement in heart failure, by at least one class, was related to the PET pattern (presence or absence of mismatch) and type of treatment (revascularization or medical therapy). More patients in the subgroup with mismatch who underwent revascularization had improvement in heart failure class.[69] Di Carli et al.[70] performed perfusion–FDG metabolism PET studies in 93 patients with left ventricular dysfunction (average LVEF, 25%); after an average follow-up of 13.6 months, 66 had severe heart failure symptoms. In the medically treated patients as a group, the severity of heart failure symptoms did not change significantly during the follow-up period. In contrast, a significant improvement in heart failure symptoms was observed only in the subgroup of patients with mismatch who underwent revascularization.[70] Stated differently, in the 34 patients with heart failure who underwent revascularization, 71% of the subgroup with a PET mismatch pattern before surgery had improvement in heart failure symptoms whereas only 31% of the patients without a PET mismatch pattern had improvement in heart failure symptoms (Fig 3).

A more recent study by Di Carli et al.[71] investigated 36 patients with ischemic cardiomyopathy (mean LVEF of 28%) who were undergoing revascularization. The preoperative extent and severity of flow-metabolism mismatch were assessed by quantitative analysis of PET images with $^{13}$N ammonia and FDG. The patients' functional status was determined before and after revascularization by using a specific activity scale. The total extent of a PET mismatch correlated linearly and significantly with the percent improvement in functional state after coronary artery bypass grafting ($r = 0.87$, $P < .0001$). A blood flow–metabolism mismatch of greater than

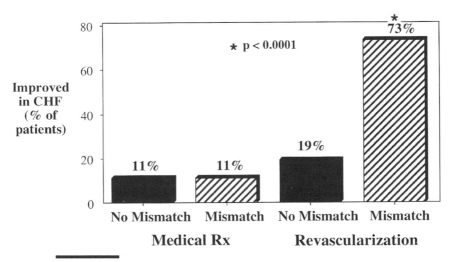

**FIGURE 3.**

Relationship between PET patterns of myocardial viability (match and mismatch), type of treatment (medical vs. myocardial revascularization), and improvement in heart failure symptoms in patients with ischemic cardiomyopathy.

18% was associated with a sensitivity of 76% and age specificity of 78% for predicting a change in functional state after revascularization. Patients with large mismatches (>18%) achieved a significantly higher functional state than those with minimal or no PET mismatch (<5%).

These data suggest that the PET pattern of myocardial viability not only predicts recovery of regional and global left ventricular dysfunction after myocardial revascularization but also identifies the subgroup of patients with poor left ventricular function and heart failure who are most likely to show relief of heart failure symptoms as a result of revascularization. Furthermore, in patients with ischemic cardiomyopathy, the magnitude of improvement in heart failure symptoms after coronary bypass surgery is related to the preoperative extent and magnitude of myocardial viability as assessed by PET imaging. Patients with large perfusion-metabolism mismatches exhibit the greatest clinical benefit after revascularization.

## POSITRON EMISSION TOMOGRAPHY PREDICTS THE POTENTIAL FOR IMPROVEMENT IN SURVIVAL AFTER REVASCULARIZATION

A major goal of noninvasive diagnostic procedures in the assessment of CAD is to evaluate the prognosis and assess the potential of a survival benefit from a treatment plan. Since survival of patients with left ventricular dysfunction relates to the resting LVEF, it may be implied that perfusion–FDG metabolism PET imaging, by predicting improvement in LVEF, also predicts survival after myocardial revascularization. This hypothesis has been addressed by two reports using perfusion–FDG metabolism PET imaging.

Eitzman et al.[69] evaluated the survival of 82 patients with left ventricular dysfunction during an average follow-up period of 12 months. Of the 44 patients who demonstrated the PET pattern of mismatch, 18 underwent medical therapy, and 26 were revascularized. Of the remaining 38 patients who did not have the PET pattern of mismatch, 24 underwent medical therapy and 14 were revascularized. Table 6 summarizes cardiac mortality in the four subgroups and shows that the highest mortality (33%) was noted in the subgroup with PET mismatch who underwent medical therapy. The mortality rate was significantly lower in patients with the PET mismatch pattern who were revascularized. Di Carli et al.[70] evaluated the survival of 93 patients with left ventricular dysfunction (average LVEF, 25%) during an average follow-up period of 13.6 months. Patients were categorized into four subgroups based

**TABLE 6.**

Relationship Between Perfusion-Metabolism Positron Emission Tomography Patterns of Myocardial Viability, Type of Treatment, and Mortality in Patients With Coronary Artery Disease and Left Ventricular Dysfunction*

| Author | N | Patients With Mismatch | | Patients Without Mismatch | |
|---|---|---|---|---|---|
| | | Med† | Rev | Med | Rev |
| Eitzman,[69] 1992 | 83 | 33%‡ (6/18) | 4% (1/26) | 8% (2/24) | 0% (0/14) |
| Di Carli,[70] 1994 | 93 | 41% (7/17) | 12% (3/26) | 9% (3/33) | 6% (1/17) |

*From Maddahi J, Schelbert HS, Brunken R, et al: *J Nucl Med* 35:707–715, 1994. Used by permission.
†Med = medical therapy; Rev = myocardial revascularization.
‡Percentages represent mortality rates during the follow-up period.

on the presence or absence of the PET mismatch pattern and the type of treatment (medical therapy vs. myocardial revascularization). As shown in Table 6, the findings were similar to those of Eitzman and associates in that the subgroup with the PET pattern of mismatch who were receiving medical therapy had the highest mortality rate, 41%. Of note, in the subgroup of patients with the PET pattern of mismatch who underwent revascularization, the mortality rate was significantly lower at 12%.

In the study of Di Carli et al.,[70] univariate analysis indicated that the extent of mismatch was the only predictor of survival. Heart failure class, chromic obstructive pulmonary disease, sex, age, prior myocardial infarction, the presence of Q waves on the resting electrocardiogram, diabetes, hypertension, the presence of angina, LVEF, extent of PET match, and revascularization were not predictors of survival in the univariate analysis. A stepwise Cox model analysis was performed to determine the prognostic contribution of mismatch when covariates with borderline significance in the univariate analysis were included in the model. The extent of mismatch and revascularization were the only predictors of survival. The relative risk (hazard) of cardiac death associated with mismatch increased by 3.5% with each unit of increment in the percent extent of mismatch, i.e., the more extensive the mismatch, the higher the risk of dying during the follow-up period. In contrast, revascularization was associated with a positive effect on survival: a decrease in the risk of cardiac death by 28%. These data

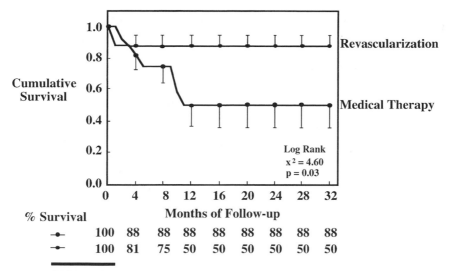

**FIGURE 4.**

Cumulative survival of 43 patients with ischemic cardiomyopathy and the PET mismatch pattern. Patients are subgrouped according to the type of treatment; revascularization (n = 17) or medical therapy (n = 17). (From Di Carli M, Davidson M, Little R, et al: *Am J Cardiol* 73:527–533, 1994. Used by permission.)

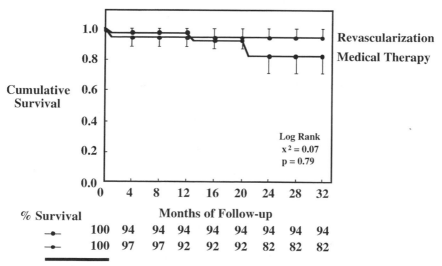

**FIGURE 5.**

Cumulative survival of 50 patients with ischemic cardiomyopathy without the PET mismatch pattern. Patients are subgrouped according to the type of treatment: revascularization (n = 33) or medical therapy (n = 17). (From Di Carli M, Davidson M, Little R, et al: *Am J Cardiol* 73:527–533, 1994. Used by permission.)

were further analyzed to assess the value of mismatch for risk stratification of patients receiving medical therapy and myocardial revascularization by using a life-table analysis. Figures 4 and 5 show
that the estimated annual survival of patients with mismatch was
lower than that of patients without mismatch (log-rank test, P =
.007). Furthermore, the annual survival probability of patients
without a mismatch was similar between the revascularized and
medical therapy subgroups.

## COST-EFFECTIVENESS OF POSITRON EMISSION TOMOGRAPHY IN THE MANAGEMENT OF CANDIDATES FOR HEART TRANSPLANTATION

Cardiac transplantation has been the ultimate therapy for end-stage
heart failure; however, because of the limited number of available
donor hearts, the waiting period for a heart transplant by eligible
recipients has been prolonged and ranges from 8 months to 2 years.
By detecting the presence of a sufficient amount of viable (hibernating) myocardium, potential candidates for myocardial revascularization may be identified. Such an approach not only lowers the
number of patients who are waiting for a transplant but also reduces the overall cost of patient care by offering coronary artery
bypass surgery to patients who would otherwise undergo cardiac
transplantation, which is more costly. In a recent study, Duong et
al.[72] evaluated 112 candidates for cardiac transplantation with
ischemic cardiomyopathy (LVEF, ≤35%) who also underwent [13]N
ammonia and FDG PET imaging for assessment of the presence and
extent of myocardial viability (hibernating myocardium). Thirty of
112 patients were found to have evidence of flow-metabolism mismatch in 2 regions of the myocardium and also had suitable coronary targets. All 30 of these patients were subsequently taken off
the transplant list and underwent coronary artery bypass graft
(CABG) surgery. The operative mortality was 10%, and 2 more patients died later in the follow-up period, for an overall mortality
rate of 16.7%. Of the remaining 82 patients who had either minimal or no evidence of PET mismatch, 33 patients underwent cardiac transplantation and 49 continued medical therapy. The perioperative mortality for cardiac transplantation was 6.1%, and 4 additional patients died during the follow-up period for an overall
mortality rate of 18.2% for patients undergoing cardiac transplantation. Of the 49 patients who underwent medical therapy, 22 patients died, a 44.9% mortality rate. The 5-year actuarial survival
rates for the CABG, transplant, and medical therapy groups were

71.4%, 80.1%, and 42.4%, respectively. Therefore, in this study, PET assessment of myocardial viability in cardiac transplant candidates allowed the identification of adequate hibernating tissue in 27% of the patients, who were subsequently referred for CABG surgery with similar perioperative and long-term survival rates as those who were referred to cardiac transplantation. In these 112 patients, use of a PET-based algorithm for the management of ischemic cardiomyopathy resulted in $3.8 million in savings in overall patient care, primarily by identifying candidates in whom coronary artery bypass surgery could be offered as an alternative to the more costly cardiac transplantation procedure.

## SUMMARY AND CONCLUSIONS

Rational management of patients with CAD and poor left ventricular function relies on proper identification of the subgroup at high risk and those who have the highest potential of benefiting from a particular type of treatment. It is now well recognized that patients with CAD and left ventricular dysfunction have a high but variable mortality rate while receiving medical therapy. Many of these patients who have intractable heart failure are considered candidates for cardiac transplantation. Despite favorable survival after cardiac transplantation, this procedure cannot be performed in 90% of the heart failure patients who are potentially eligible because of the shortage of donor hearts. Cardiac transplantation is also an expensive procedure. Perfusion–FDG metabolism PET imaging has become the gold-standard noninvasive imaging method to identify the presence and extent of hibernating myocardium. Positron emission tomography accurately predicts recovery of regional and global left ventricular dysfunction after revascularization. In patients with poor left ventricular function, the PET pattern of perfusion metabolism mismatch is also predictive of improvement in heart failure symptoms and survival benefit after myocardial revascularization. These data suggest that a rational approach may be developed for cost-effective management of patients with CAD and poor left ventricular function.

### ACKNOWLEDGMENT

The authors are grateful to Sepehr Rokhsar and Amiel Balagtas for their research assistance, to Terri Meredith for preparation of this manuscript, and to Diane Martin for preparing the figures.

# REFERENCES

1. Oberman A, Jones W, Riley C, et al: Natural history of coronary artery disease. *Bull N Y Acad Med* 48:1109, 1972.
2. Bruschke A, Proudfit W, Sones F: Progress study of 490 consecutive nonsurgical cases of coronary disease followed 5–9 years. II. Ventriculographic and other correlations. *Circulation* 47:1154, 1973.
3. Yatteau R, Peter R, Behar V: Ischemic cardiomyopathy: The myopathy of coronary artery disease. *Am J Cardiol* 34:520–525, 1974.
4. Nelson G, Cohn P, Gorlin R: Prognosis in medically-treated coronary artery disease: Influence of ejection fraction compared to other parameters. *Circulation* 52:408–412, 1975.
5. Manley J, King J, Zeft J, et al: The "bad" left ventricle; results of coronary surgery and effect on later survival. *J Thorac Cardiovasc Surg* 72:841–848, 1976.
6. Parker J: Prognosis in coronary artery disease. *Clev Clin Q* 45:145–146, 1978.
7. Faulkner S, Stoney W, Alford W, et al: Ischemic cardiomyopathy: Medical versus surgical treatment. *J Thorac Cardiovasc Surg* 74:77–82, 1977.
8. Harris P, Phil D, Harrell F, et al: Survival in medically treated coronary artery disease. *Circulation* 60:1259–1269, 1979.
9. Franciosa J, Wilen M, Ziesche S, et al: Survival in men with severe chronic left ventricular failure due to either coronary heart disease or idiopathic dilated cardiomyopathy. *Am J Cardiol* 51:831–836, 1983.
10. Alderman E, Fisher L, Litwin P: Results of coronary artery surgery in patients with poor left ventricular function (CASS). *Circulation* 4:788–795, 1983.
11. Killip T, Passamani E, Davis K, et al: Coronary artery surgery study (CASS): A randomized trial of coronary bypass surgery. *Circulation* 72(suppl 5):102–109, 1985.
12. CASS V: Eleven-year survival in the Veterans Administration randomized trial of coronary bypass surgery for stable angina. *N Engl J Med* 311:1333–1339, 1984.
13. Mock M, Ringqvist I, Fisher L, et al: Survival of medically treated patients in the coronary artery surgery study (CASS) registry. *Circulation* 66:562–568, 1982.
14. Pigott J, Kouchoukos N, Oberman A, et al: Late results of surgical and medical therapy for patients with coronary artery disease and depressed left ventricular function. *J Am Coll Cardiol* 5:1036–1045, 1985.
15. Bounous E, Mark D, Pollock B, et al: Surgical survival benefits for coronary disease patients with left ventricular dysfunction. *Circulation* 78(suppl 1):151–157, 1988.
16. Van Trigt P: Ischemic cardiomyopathy: The role of coronary artery bypass. *Coron Artery Dis* 4:707–712, 1993.

17. Califf R, Harrell F, Lee K, et al: The evolution of medical and surgical therapy for coronary artery disease. *JAMA* 261:2077–2086, 1989.
18. Luciani G, Faggian G, Mazzucco A, et al: Myocardial revascularization in ischemic cardiomyopathy: A way for better donor heart allocation. *Transplant Proc* 25:3137–3174, 1993.
19. Luciani G, Faggian G, Razzolini R, et al: Severe ischemic left ventricular failure: Coronary operation or heart transplantation? *Ann Thorac Surg* 55:719–723, 1993.
20. Evans R, Manninen D, Garrison L, et al: Donor availability as the primary determinant of the future of heart transplantation. *JAMA* 255:1982–1988, 1986.
21. Cohn P, Gorlin R, Cohn L, et al: Left ventricular ejection fraction as a prognosis guide in surgical treatment of coronary and valvular heart disease. *Am J Cardiol* 34:136–141, 1974.
22. Kennedy J, Kaiser G, Fisher L, et al: Clinical and angiographic predictors of operative mortality from the collaborative study in coronary artery surgery (CASS) 1. *Circulation* 63:793–802, 1981.
23. Freeman A, Walshhi W, Giles R: Early and long-term results of coronary artery bypass grafting with severely depressed left ventricular performance. *Am J Cardiol* 54:749–754, 1984.
24. Dreyfus G, Duboc D, Blasco A, et al: Myocardial viability assessment in ischemic cardiomyopathy: Benefits of coronary revascularization. *Ann Thorac Surg* 57:1402–1408, 1994.
25. Elefteriades J, Tolis G Jr, Levi E, et al: Coronary artery bypass grafting in severe left ventricular dysfunction: Excellent survival with improved ejection fraction and functional state. *J Am Coll Cardiol* 22:1411–1417, 1993.
26. Christakis G, Wesiel R, Fremes S, et al: Coronary artery bypass grafting in patients with poor ventricular function. *J Thorac Cardiovasc Surg* 103:1083–1092, 1992.
27. Kron I, Flanagan T, Balckbourne L: Coronary revascularization rather than cardiac transplantation for chronic ischemic cardiomyopathy. *Ann Surg* 210:348–352, 1989.
28. Tyras D, Kaiser G, Barner H, et al: Global left ventricular impairment and myocardial revascularization: Determinants of survival. *Ann Thorac Surg* 37:47–51, 1984.
29. Coles J, Del Campo C, Ahmed S, et al: Improved long-term survival following myocardial revascularization in patients with severe left ventricular dysfunction. *J Thorac Cardiovasc Surg* 81:846–850, 1981.
30. Mitchel B, Alivizatos P, Adam M, et al: Myocardial revascularization in patients with poor ventricular function. *J Thorac Cardiovasc Surg* 69:52–62, 1975.
31. Hung J, Kelly D, Baird D, et al: Aorta-coronary bypass grafting in patients with severe left ventricular dysfunction. *J Thorac Cardiovasc Surg* 79:718–723, 1980.

32. Hochberg M, Parsonnet V, Gielchinski I, et al: Coronary artery bypass grafting in patients with ejection fractions below forty percent. *J Thorac Cardiovasc Surg* 86:519–527, 1983.
33. Louie H, Laks H, Milgalter E: Ischemic cardiomyopathy: Criteria for coronary revascularization and cardiac transplantation. *Circulation* 84(suppl 3):290–295, 1991.
34. Passamani E, Davis K, Gillespie M: A randomized trial of coronary artery bypass surgery: Survival of patients with a low ejection fraction. *N Engl J Med* 312:1665–1671, 1985.
35. Isom O, Spencer F, Glassman E, et al: Long-term survival following coronary bypass surgery in patients with significant impairment of left ventricular function. *Circulation* 52(suppl 1):141–147, 1979.
36. Wechsler A, Junod F: Coronary bypass grafting in patients with chronic congestive heart failure. *Circulation* 79(suppl 1):92–96, 1989.
37. Rahimtoola S: The hibernating myocardium. *Am Heart J* 117:211–221, 1989.
38. Rahimtoola S: A perspective on the three large multicenter randomized clinical trials of coronary bypass surgery for chronic stable angina. *Circulation* 72(suppl 5):123–135, 1985.
39. Braunwald E, Kloner R: The stunned myocardium: Prolonged, postischemic ventricular dysfunction. *Circulation* 66:1146–1149, 1982.
40. Schelbert H, Phelps M, Hoffman E: Regional myocardial perfusion assessed with N-13 labeled ammonia and positron emission computerized axial tomography. *Am J Cardiol* 43:209–218, 1979.
41. Schelbert H, Phelps M, Huang S: N-13 ammonia as an indicator of myocardial blood flow. *Circulation* 63:1259–1272, 1981.
42. Gould K, Schelbert H, Phelps M, et al: Noninvasive assessment of coronary stenoses with myocardial perfusion imaging during pharmacologic coronary vasodilation. V. Detection of 47 percent diameter coronary stenosis with intravenous nitrogen-13 ammonia and emission-computed transaxial tomography in intact dogs. *Am J Cardiol* 43:200–208, 1979.
43. Mullani N, Goldstein R, Gould K: Perfusion imaging with rubidium-82: I. Measurement of extraction and flow with external detectors. *J Nucl Med* 24:898–906, 1983.
44. Bergmann S, Fox K, Rand A: Quantification of regional myocardial blood flow in vivo with $H_2^{15}O$. *Circulation* 70:724–733, 1984.
45. Bergmann S, Herrero P, Markham J: Noninvasive quantitation of myocardial blood flow in human subjects with oxygen-15–labeled water and positron emission tomography. *J Am Coll Cardiol* 14:639–652, 1989.
46. Araujo L, Lammertsma A, Rhodes E: Noninvasive quantification of regional myocardial blood flow in coronary artery disease with oxygen-15–labeled carbon dioxide inhalation and positron emission tomography. *Circulation* 83:875–885, 1991.
47. Phelps M, Hoffman E, Selin C: Investigation of [$^{18}$F] 2-fluoro-2-

deoxyglucose for the measure of myocardial glucose metabolism. *J Nucl Med* 19:1311–1319, 1978.

48. Sokoloff L, Reivich M, Kennedy D, et al: The [$^{14}$C] deoxyglucose method for the measurement of local cerebral glucose utilization: Theory, procedure and normal values in the conscious and anesthetized albino rat. *J Neurochem* 28:897–916, 1977.

49. Ratib O, Phelps M, Huang S: Positron tomography with deoxyglucose for estimating local myocardial glucose metabolism. *J Nucl Med* 23:577–586, 1982.

50. Choi Y, Brunken R, Hawkins R: Factors affecting myocardial 2-[F-18] fluoro-2-deoxy-D-glucose uptake in positron emission tomography studies of normal humans. *Eur J Nucl Med* 20:308–318, 1993.

51. Berry J, Baker J, Pieper K: The effect of metabolic milieu on cardiac PET imaging using fluorine-18-deoxyglucose and nitrogen-13-ammonia in normal volunteers. *J Nucl Med* 32:1518–1525, 1991.

52. Marshall R, Tillisch J, Phelps M: Identification and differentiation of resting myocardial ischemia and infarction in man with positron computed tomography $^{18}$F-labeled fluorodeoxyglucose and N-13 ammonia. *Circulation* 67:766–778, 1983.

53. Camici P, Araujo L, Spinks T: Increased uptake of $^{18}$F-fluorodeoxyglucose in postischemic myocardium of patients with exercise-induced angina. *Circulation* 74:81–88, 1986.

54. Opie L: Effects of regions ischemia on metabolism of glucose and fatty acids: Relative rate of aerobic and anaerobic energy production during myocardial infarction and comparison with effects of anoxia. *Circ Res* 38(suppl 1):52–74, 1976.

55. Opie L: Myocardial ischemia—metabolic pathways and implications of increased glycolysis. *Cardio Drugs Ther* 4:777–790, 1990.

56. Tamaki N, Ohtani H, Yamashita K: Metabolic activity in the areas of new fill-in after thallium-201 reinjection: Comparison with positron emission tomography using fluorine-18-deoxyglucose. *J Nucl Med* 31:457, 1991.

57. Tillisch J, Brunken R, Marshall R: Reversibility of cardiac wall-motion abnormalities predicted by positron tomography. *N Engl J Med* 314:884–888, 1986.

58. Tamaki N, Yonekura Y, Yamashita K: Positron emission tomography using fluorine-18-deoxyglucose in evaluation of coronary artery bypass grafting. *Am J Cardiol* 64:860–865, 1989.

59. Lucignani G, Paolini G, Landoni C: Presurgical identification of hibernating myocardium by combined use of technetium-99m hexakis 2-methoxyisobutylisonitrile single photon emission tomography and fluorine-18-fluoro-2-deoxy-D-glucose positron emission tomography in patients with coronary artery disease. *Eur J Nucl Med* 19:874–881, 1992.

60. Carrel T, Jenni R, Haubold-Reuter S: Improvement of severely reduced left ventricular function after surgical revascularization in patients

       with preoperative myocardial infarction. *Eur J Cardiothorac Surg* 6:479–484, 1992.

61. Gropler R, Siegel B, Sampathkumaran K: Dependence of recovery of contractile function on maintenance of oxidative metabolism after myocardial infarction. *J Am Cardiol* 19:989–997, 1992.

62. Gropler R, Geltman E, Sampathkumaran K: Comparison of carbon-11-acetate with fluorine-18-fluorodeoxyglucose for delineating viable myocardium by positron emission tomography. *J Am Coll Cardiol* 22:1587–1597, 1993.

63. Paolini G, Lucignani G, Zuccari M, et al: Identification and revascularization of hibernating myocardium in angina-free patients with left ventricular dysfunction. *Eur J Cardiothorac Surg* 8:139–144, 1994.

64. Marwick T, MacIntyre W, Lafont A: Metabolic responses of hibernating and infarcted myocardium to revascularization: A follow-up study of regional perfusion, function, and metabolism. *Circulation* 85:1347–1353, 1992.

65. Knuuti M, Nuutila P, Ruotsalainen U: The value of quantitative analysis of glucose utilization in detection of myocardial viability by PET. *J Nucl Med* 34:2068–2075, 1993.

66. vom Dahl J, Altehoefer C, Sheehan F: Myocardial viability assessed by combined nuclear imaging using myocardial scintigraphy and positron emission tomography: Impact on treatment and functional outcome following revascularization. *J Am Coll Cardiol* 1995, in press.

67. Besozzi M, Brown M, Hubner K: Retrospective post therapy evaluation of cardiac function in 208 coronary artery disease patients evaluated by positron emission tomography (abstract). *J Nucl Med* 33:885, 1992.

68. Depre C, Melin J, Vanoverschelde J: Assessment of myocardial viability after bypass surgery by pre-operative PET flow-metabolism measurements and ultrastructural analysis of myocardial biopsies (abstract). *Circulation* 88(suppl 1):199, 1993.

69. Eitzman D, Al-Aouar Z, Kanter H: Clinical outcome of patients with advanced coronary artery disease after viability studies with positron emission tomography. *J Am Coll Cardiol* 20:559–565, 1992.

70. Di Carli M, Davidson M, Little R, et al: Value of metabolic imaging with positron emission tomography for evaluating prognosis in patients with coronary artery disease and left ventricular dysfunction. *Am J Cardiol* 73:527–533, 1994.

71. Di Carli M, Asgarzadie F, Schelbert H, et al: Quantitative relation between myocardial viability and improvement in heart failure symptoms after revascularization in patients with ischemic cardiomyopathy. *Circulation* 1995, in press.

72. Duong T, Hendi P, Fonarow G, et al: Role of positron emission tomographic assessment of myocardial viability in the management of patients who are referred for cardiac transplantation. *Circulation* 1995, in press.

# Index